HOLISTIC KETO FOR GUT HEALTH

"Western medicine has shown its value in diagnosing and treating disease but is often lacking in explaining the origins of autoimmune and inflammatory disease states—specifically the role the gastrointestinal system plays in maintaining homeostasis. In her book *Holistic Keto for Gut Health* Kristin Grayce McGary bridges the gap between conventional and holistic medicine while staying true to her scientific roots; she clearly has a mastery of her field. Many of my patients would benefit from understanding the topics covered in this book."

— AARON LEE, MD, doctor of gastroenterology

"In a world of fad diets and nutritional confusion, Kristin Grayce McGary provides a fresh new insight into the role of nutrition in health and healing. Her nutrition recommendations are grounded in science and the latest research into the gut microbiome. If you suffer from any chronic illness or autoimmune disease and are struggling in the world of conventional medicine, you need to read this book. It has the potential to accelerate your journey to optimal health."

— NAUMAN NAEEM, MD, author of *Healing from the Inside Out*

"Kristin Grayce McGary has identified the problems that underpin poor health and immunity and offers solutions. Offering cutting-edge ideas combined with common sense and delicious recipes, *Holistic Keto for Gut Health* is a must-read if you suffer from any type of chronic condition. McGary is an impressive author with good clinical sense and a pioneer in her field. Highly recommended!"

— SUZY COHEN, RPh, America's Most Trusted Pharmacist®
and author of *Drug Muggers*

"This book could save your life! *Holistic Keto for Gut Health* is an authoritative text combined with tasty recipes that teaches you how to use food as medicine. I'm grateful to have such a comprehensive guidebook as a personal resource as well as to share with all of my students and clients."

— DARREN R. WEISSMAN, D.C, developer of the LifeLine Technique
and author of *Awakening to the Secret Code of Your Mind*

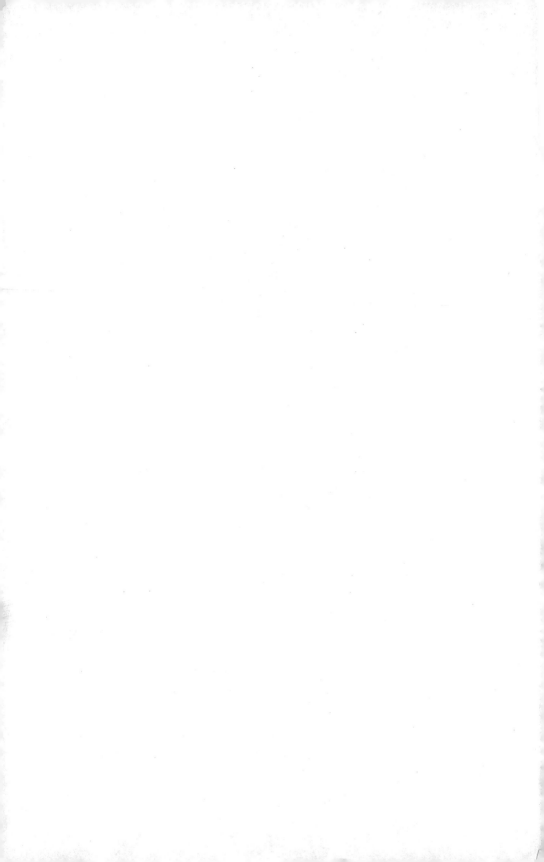

**A PROGRAM FOR RESETTING
YOUR METABOLISM**

HOLISTIC
KETO
FOR GUT HEALTH

Kristin Grayce McGary

LAc., MAc., CFMP®, CST-T, CLP,
Health and Lifestyle Alchemist

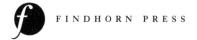 FINDHORN PRESS

Findhorn Press
One Park Street
Rochester, Vermont 05767
www.findhornpress.com

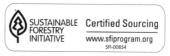

Text stock is SFI certified

Findhorn Press is a division of Inner Traditions International

Disclaimer

The information in this book is given in good faith and is neither intended
to diagnose any physical or mental condition nor to serve as a substitute for
informed medical advice or care. Please contact your health professional
for medical advice and treatment. Neither author nor publisher can be
held liable by any person for any loss or damage whatsoever which may
arise from the use of this book or any of the information therein.

Any product names, brands, and other trademarks featured or referred
to within the book are the property of their respective trademark holders.
The material in this book reflects the opinions of the author, not the
respective trademark holders. The author is neither affiliated with
nor sponsored, approved, or endorsed by Cyrex Laboratories
or any other brand or company mentioned in this book.

Cataloging-in-Publication data for this title
is available from the Library of Congress

ISBN 978-1-62055-981-9 (print)
ISBN 978-1-62055-982-6 (ebook)

Printed and bound in the United States by Lake Book Manufacturing, Inc.
The text stock is SFI certified. The Sustainable Forestry Initiative®
program promotes sustainable forest management.

10 9 8 7 6 5 4 3 2 1

Edited by Nicky Leach
Photographs from pixabay.com
Text design and layout by Anna-Kristina Larsson
This book was typeset in Montserrat and Aleo

To send correspondence to the author of this book,
mail a first-class letter to the author c/o Inner Traditions ·
Bear & Company, One Park Street, Rochester, VT 05767, USA
and we will forward the communication, or contact the
author directly at **www.kristingraycemcgary.com**

To Greg, my incredible husband, who has selflessly and compassionately empowered me to follow my heart. He has loved me like no other, and even appreciates my mistakes—especially in the kitchen—and savors them all.

And to you, dear reader, for the courage it takes to change your diet and life, to find strength, creativity, self-love, and grace in a world that seems to no longer value healthy food and holistic lifestyle choices. This book is for you.

Contents

Part III: The Functional Ketogenic Gut Repair Program

Part IV: The Food

Preface

I wasn't always healthy. I was born in the Midwest in the early 1970s, where my family and community had a very limited awareness of nutrition. Thankfully, we had a garden with fresh vegetables and a memorable patch of strawberries in the backyard. But everyone in my family was overweight, some grossly so. My mom was always on and off diets like the Tomato Soup Diet, the Grapefruit Diet, and even the Microwave Diet.

By age 10, I was chubby, but fortunately, we then moved to Arizona, where I got a bicycle and joined a summer swim team. After a few weeks of swimming and riding, I had lost 10 pounds. I hardly noticed, although my bathing suit sagged embarrassingly, but eventually it was impossible not to notice the difference between my weight and health and the weight and (lack of) health exhibited by the rest of my family. By age 15, I had begun to make conscious food choices. I even began to refuse fast food on family vacations.

Until I reached 20 years of age, I strengthened athletically through dance, softball, swimming, soccer, track and field, cycling, and even competed in body building for three years. I had several coaches and a roommate who mentored me in nutrition and exercise. I was informed, strong, ripped, and always on the move. But for some reason, during my beginning years as a pre-med student at the University of Arizona and while working as an emergency medical technician (EMT), I began to experience pain, undiagnosed anemia, gas, bloating, energy crashes, and severe hypoglycemia (low blood sugar).

I tried to heal myself by, among other things, becoming a vegetarian. But my symptoms worsened, and I began to suffer from unstable body weight, episodes of debilitating pain with spasms, pain in my TMJ (temporal mandibular joint, the jaw hinge), sleep problems, brain fog, headaches, and ever-lower energy. I went to doctor after doctor, but no one could figure out what was wrong with me. I was eventually diagnosed with fibromyalgia.

All the while I kept upping my game, doing research, reading, becoming more and more health-aware and trying to fix my problems. But I was deeply frustrated and puzzled. How could someone so health-conscious feel so bad? I didn't understand what was happening to me, but I persevered in trying to find answers to my deteriorating condition.

One of my most shocking realizations was that traditional Western medicine wasn't going to give me the answers—that sporting an MD or ND behind their names didn't make men and women omniscient. It didn't make them capable of accurately understanding a patient's full health picture. It didn't guarantee that they were trained in proper diagnosis. It didn't mean that they would always order the correct lab work, or even understand and properly interpret the test results when they came back. All my doctors were well-intentioned, but that wasn't going to get me healthy.

So I changed gears and searched for solutions elsewhere, and (eventually) pursued a degree in Asian and Functional medicine. I also explored electrodermal screening, acupuncture, herbs, homeopathy, biological medicine, dark field microscopy, rapid eye movement technique, biological dentistry, flower essences, neural therapy, craniosacral therapy, somato-emotional release, nutrition, family constellation, shamanism, meditation, and chi gong—all in an ongoing effort to try to heal myself.

My independent healing work paid off. My last episode of debilitating pain was on Thanksgiving 1996, when my son was three months old. Except for occasional gut bloating and pain, all of my symptoms went away. Years later, though, I began to experience a new set of mysterious symptoms, and my quest to heal began again.

After more years of unanswered questions, I was hospitalized for severe hyponatremia (electrolyte imbalance) following an intense bladder infection and drinking too much water, which flushed out my electrolytes and caused a serious condition.

The ER doc ordered a TSH (Thyroid Stimulating Hormone) test, and it was off the charts high, an indicator that I was severely hypothyroid. I consulted a naturopath, who ordered a thyroid antibody test. Two tests showed antibody readings at 1,000 and 500 (the numbers should be zero), and I was formally diagnosed with Hashimoto's thyroiditis.

I now began what I thought would be the final chapter of my healing journey. But after several years as a lab rat, dosed with a variety of thyroid medications, iodine, nutritional changes, biological dentistry, Wilson's Temperature Syndrome Protocol—you name it—I actually felt worse, experiencing weight fluctuations, extreme hair loss, debilitating fatigue, and brain fog.

It wasn't until I learned about intestinal health and gut repair that I began to grasp that one of the roots of the autoimmunity and thyroid challenges was my gut. And it wasn't until I learned the value of a truly comprehensive lab panel, and how to interpret the results based on a healthy scale rather than the normal disease-based scale, that things actually shifted.

I researched Blood Type Diet, Macrobiotic, Metabolic Type Diet, Paleo, Primal, and Ketogenic diets; alternative thyroid medications; functional testing; subconscious patterns and beliefs; api-therapy; and stem cell therapy—at long last entering the final phase of my healing journey.

As I addressed the real causes of my problems—inflammation, unbalanced intestinal health, and sabotaging belief patterns—my antibodies dropped significantly. The awful energy crashes stopped, my weight stabilized, the razor-sharp pain in my gut disappeared, my white blood cell levels increased, and my mood improved.

I was introduced to Bee Venom Therapy (BVT), and those bees began to work their magic! The gamma hemolytic strep disappeared, and I cut my thyroid medication in half in just a few months. But then perimenopause began earlier than expected, and as my hormones changed, my beautiful thyroid become out of sorts again. And the journey continued.

Today, I'm another person. I'm a healthy, strong, vibrant woman and a health professional. I've explored dozens of eating programs designed to address intestinal health and inflammation and found benefits and harm in them all. In addition, I've done an immense amount of research into diet, gut health, and autoimmune diseases. I've worked with hundreds of patients suffering as I once did and have helped them regain their health. And I've hit upon a ketogenic-type diet with an added emphasis on gut repair that works. I continue to learn and share information with my community. If you'd like to join me please sign up for my complimentary newsletter, filled with recipes and clinical pearls to keep you informed, empowered, healthy, and vibrant: www.kristingraycemcgary.com

The program I share with you in this book changed my life—and probably saved it. And it's changed (and possibly saved) the lives of many others whose gastrointestinal tracts had been damaged by decades of processed foods, stress, toxic chemical exposures, hidden food sensitivities, and unhealthy lifestyles. Now I pass the information on to you.

Introduction

Do you feel exhausted and experience foggy thinking and other mysterious symptoms that come and go? Symptoms your doctors can't figure out, and yet they keep prescribing more and more medications to suppress the symptoms?

Do you have headaches or migraines, sinus congestion, or allergies? Do you have digestive troubles such as gas, bloating, diarrhea, constipation, acid reflux, irritable bowel syndrome (IBS), irritable bowel disease (IBD), stomach pain, and weight gain or sudden weight loss? Do you suffer from joint pain and stiffness, hair loss, brittle nails, dry skin, sleep challenges, hormone imbalances, diabetes, insulin resistance, diabetes, metabolic syndrome, cardiovascular disease, skin problems such as eczema and psoriasis, thyroid dysfunction, or any other autoimmune disorder? Are you ready for answers, empowerment, and hope? Are you ready to level up your health and nutrition?

If so, this book is for you.

Your gastrointestinal health and the health of other areas of your life mutually reflect each other. Any level of gut disharmony, no matter how small, impacts other areas of your body. Meanwhile, the conditions of your life—nutrition, stress, genetic factors, hydration, trauma, and environmental factors such as toxins, pesticides, preservatives, and plastics—directly impact your gut and therefore your brain, your hormones, your immune system, your organ function, the way you think, the way you feel, and the way you cope.

This may be a new concept to you, and it may seem unfathomable that your gut possesses such wide-ranging power to influence so many corners of your life. But it does.

The American Autoimmune Related Diseases Association (AARDA) estimates that as many as 50 million Americans suffer from an autoimmune disease in which their body's immune system mistakenly attacks its own healthy tissues and cells. These include lupus, multiple sclerosis, rheumatoid arthritis, Type I diabetes mellitus, Grave's disease, psoriasis, inflammatory bowel disease (IBD), and Hashimoto's thyroiditis, just to name a few.

If this estimate is correct, the crippling epidemic of autoimmunity affects up to five times more people than cancer. The symptoms are puzzlingly broad in scope, resist accurate testing, and are poorly diagnosed, which means that many, if not most, people with an autoimmune disease suffer endless years of pain and fruitless medical interventions.

As a healthcare provider in recovery from an autoimmune disease, I've discovered the necessity of a comprehensive, compassionate, and holistic approach to healing.

The book you hold in your hands contains a gut-repair program of optimal nutrition and healthy lifestyle that reverses damage to the intestinal walls, promotes healthy flora, and supports proper nutrient absorption, elimination, immune function, hormone balance, neurotransmitter production, longevity, and vitality. It is a comprehensive program that will bring you a renewed sense of empowerment, freedom, and yes, health. This book combines elements of the Paleo, Primal, and Ketogenic diets that are specifically effective for healing the gastrointestinal tract—the seat of autoimmune issues. As a licensed Asian medical practitioner, I also include aspects of Eastern healing work. You'll also find a vast array of other ideas, protocols, and health approaches that will help you approach gut healing in a truly holistic way.

Knowledge is power. There's a lot of incomplete, inaccurate information on diet and health out there. It's important to be an informed consumer, armed with pertinent facts about gut repair and long-term gut health. This is why this comprehensive book contains fascinating information and stories. I back up everything I say with science and research. If you find yourself a little overwhelmed by some of the science, skim or skip it. You'll find all the guidance you need, and that's what matters.

What Is Health?

We've been conditioned to see health as the "absence" of disease, defect, or pain, but I believe that health means the "presence" of something—presence of lasting energy, clear thinking, good memory, healthy digestion, detoxification and excretion, muscle strength and flexibility, emotional stability, joy, and deep peace. This is the optimal healthy state of well-being.

The Old English word *haelp* meant "wholeness, being whole, sound, or well." The Proto-German word *hailitho* also means "whole." Old Norse offers *helge*, meaning "holy, sacred." This "wholeness" refers to all of your vital parts and processes as present, properly arranged, and in harmonious balance.[1]

Basically, there are two dimensions to wholeness: physical and energetic. The physical dimension includes anatomy, biochemistry, and biological processes. The energetic dimension includes the awareness that integrates body, mind, and emotion. Both are necessary for healing and optimal health.

Another point I want to make upfront is that **food is medicine**.

Food impacts you biochemically and either enhances or hinders the performance of your bodily systems. Just as a pharmaceutical drug has a biochemical structure that has specific effects on the body, so do the many chemical components of foods. What you eat matters. When choosing foods, you need to consider more than flavor, calorie count, or a balance of protein, fat, and carbohydrate. You need to nourish all dimensions of your being: physiological, neurological, psychological, emotional, and spiritual. This book will guide you through proven methods.

Learn to listen to your body, become informed, and consult a holistic, integrative, and functional healthcare provider with any questions and concerns.

PART I

Why Ketogenic Gut Repair?

Chapter 1

Autoimmunity, Your Gut, and Your Other Brain

You've probably heard the maxim "You are what you eat." The truth is closer to this, "You are what you digest and absorb."

Most people in developed nations consume grains, gluten, milk, eggs, processed foods, trans-fats, preservatives, food colorings, non-organics, soy, corn, buckets of sugar, and increasing amounts of genetically modified foods. We're exposed to hundreds of toxic chemicals, pesticides, herbicides, paints, sealers, glues, and heavy metals through our air, water, food, and body care products. We endure incredible burdens of stress in a culture ever more obsessed with speed and consumption. We don't just want fast food but also instant medical treatments, get-rich-quick business deals, rapid promotions, turbo-charged cars, hyper-passionate relationships, dramatic detoxification programs, power yoga, and even instant enlightenment!

All this impacts your health and well-being, especially your gastrointestinal health, impairing the gut's capacity to absorb nutrients and resulting in undernourishment (even as you overeat), which contributes even more stress.

The gut is the throne of immune function. The complex enteric nervous system (ENS, often referred to as the "second brain"), located in your gut, is vital in that it affects every aspect of your physical, emotional, and psychological health. If there's any imbalance, your body is compromised, and you will suffer in some way, eventually. Bottom line: If you're alive on the planet today, your gut is under attack, and the epidemic of autoimmunity and autoimmune disease, cancer, and allergies in the world today is proof.

These are all symptoms of immune dysfunction. Autoimmunity occurs when your immune system is misdirected and attacks your body by making antibodies against your own tissues. According to the National Institutes of Health Autoimmune Diseases Coordinating Committee, autoimmune disease is on the rise. Approximately 24 million Americans, 8 percent of the population, are thought to suffer from an autoimmune disease. By way of context, "cancer affected approximately 9 million people and heart disease affected approximately 22 million people in the United States."[2]

The estimate of 24 million people with autoimmune disease is half that of the American Autoimmune Related Diseases Association. It is likely a huge underestimate, because our healthcare system usually fails to diagnose an autoimmune disease until signs and symptoms (including out-of-range lab markers) indicate significant irreversible damage to organs, glands, and tissue has already occurred.

Symptoms of immune and gut dysfunction are ubiquitous and rarely correctly identified:

- Hypersensitivity to specific foods or environmental allergens such as pollens, perfumes, toxins, and cleaning products. These often appear prior to a full-blown autoimmune disease.
- Digestive disorders such as constipation, diarrhea, gas, bloating, excess weight, abdominal or stomach pain or discomfort, gastroesophageal reflux disease (GERD or acid reflux), irritable bowel syndrome (IBS) or irritable bowel disease (IBD), and blood or mucus in your stools are so common, few doctors relate them to autoimmunity.
- Recurrent infections, joint and muscle pain and swelling, rheumatoid arthritis, cancer, lupus, scleroderma, Hashimoto's thyroiditis, type 1 diabetes, immune dysfunction disorder (also known as chronic fatigue syndrome), and Epstein Barr virus (EBV) are also autoimmunity and gut problem indicators that usually end up not being treated at the level of gut function.

Which means the number of people affected in the U.S. is realistically closer to 72 million—nearly a quarter of the U.S. population.

Even something as simple (and unobvious) as not having a strong fever accompanying a cold or flu for more than three years is a sign. Yes, fevers are usually a sign of health. Why? For one thing, it means your immune system is working well enough to mount a vigorous response to infection. On the other hand, a low-grade, recurrent fever may be a sign of an autoimmune disease, Lyme disease, or cancer, and is completely different from the strong fever you get at the onset of a cold or flu. The *absence* of strong fever for many years often means your immune system is weak or out of balance.

Getting sick can be a healthy workout for your immune system. Plus, a fever is a natural anti-cancer, detoxifying, immune-stimulating event. When your body temperature is about four degrees higher than normal (98.6°F is normal), your white blood cell count increases tenfold, and white blood cells are an important part of your immune function—they go after the bad guys, destroy them, then clean up.

This is one reason more and more cancer centers are incorporating far-infrared sauna technology into treatment plans for their patients. Far-infrared can increase core body temperature, stimulating the immune system in a balanced way and increasing metabolism and healthy detoxification. Think of a far-infrared sauna as a tool for externally inducing a fever.

The Immune System: A Little Background

The development of immune dysfunction and an autoimmune disease is influenced by three factors: genetic vulnerability, immune system response to environmental exposures (such as toxic chemicals, antigenic foods, infectious agents), and gut health (intestinal permeability).

Nutrition; lifestyle; pharmaceuticals, such as antibiotics, non-steroidal anti-inflammatory drugs (NSAIDs), including aspirin and ibuprofen, antacids, proton pump inhibitors and histamine 2 blockers; environmental factors, such as toxins, heavy metals, pesticides; and pathogens, such as viruses, bacteria, parasites, and fungi that damage tissue and trigger genetic mutations and epigenetic influences, all lead to gastrointestinal damage, inflammation, and immune dysregulation.

Stress can cause a cascade of endocrine and immune-system dysregulation that can amplify autoimmunity into an autoimmune disease pattern. It also causes unhealthy fluctuations in cortisol, the so-called "stress hormone." Long-distance sports often create an imbalance in cortisol, as does exercising in the evening or working the nighttime "graveyard shift."

Autoimmune disease is mostly preventable, but appropriate testing and accurate interpretation of test results are essential. Immune dysfunction can be easily identified through functional blood chemistry analysis of a comprehensive blood panel. But it's essential to know what to test and how to read it appropriately. For example, I see patients weekly who have low levels of thyroid antibodies, indicating autoimmunity, but no one has ever tested them or educated them about what this may mean for their health. In fact, many Western doctors consider low-level thyroid antibodies as "normal."

In the United States, Hashimoto's autoimmune thyroiditis is considered the most prevalent autoimmune disorder.[3] Hashimoto's has been identified as the mechanism behind hypothyroidism in 90 percent of cases.[4] One study has shown that thyroid antibodies are a marker for future thyroid disease.[5] So I always want to see thyroid antibodies on every comprehensive lab, regardless of symptoms. Yet blood panels are often misread or not done at all, and symptoms are ignored or misidentified.

I see many people in my practice with autoimmunity who haven't yet sustained sufficient tissue damage or had antibody levels elevated enough to receive a diagnosis. They don't yet have a traditionally diagnosable autoimmune disease. This is both good and bad. It's great that it hasn't moved into a severe disease pattern and can be easily halted. But it's not great to have such severe immune dysfunction that your body is attacking itself in the first place.

It doesn't take long for chemical exposure, genetic predisposition, nutritional exposures to foods such as gluten and dairy, or a severe stressor to push your system into a full-blown autoimmune disease state. But who wants things to progress that far? If someone had done this level of comprehensive testing and healthcare for me when I began suffering, it would have saved me thousands of dollars and many years of pain!

Case Study

"Suzy" was 52 years young when we first met, the mother of two teenagers and a fitness professional. For more than a year, she didn't believe it was necessary to run a comprehensive lab panel because her doctor had run a few labs and said everything was fine. She had many autoimmune symptoms but thought that things would change on their own. She was often fatigued; had cloudy thinking; depended on sugar, caffeine, and carbohydrates for energy; and had painful, often swollen joints, especially after eating gluten. She had a history of chronic digestive problems like gas, bloating, and constipation. She also had chronic sinus congestion and reported going into perimenopause at age 40 and menopause at age 50.

After a few years of suffering, she came to see me specifically to have her comprehensive lab panel analyzed. She'd been under the care of a Western MD and a naturopath for years and been put on a thyroid medication because her thyroid-stimulating hormone (TSH) was elevated. But no other thyroid tests had been ordered.

This was unfathomable to me. There are eight markers of thyroid function and two antibody tests that I always need to see in order to accurately determine the root of any thyroid disorder. This lovely lady had been put on a thyroid drug without ever having a full panel of thyroid tests to see if the treatment was even appropriate!

How could this happen? Simple: MDs are bound to follow standard of care protocols that dictate how doctors must respond to lab results. If you have elevated TSH, the standard of care prescribes treatment with a T4 drug, often synthetic and often inappropriate.

After 10 years of taking this medication and enduring symptoms that interrupted her life and relationships, we discovered that she suffered from Hashimoto's thyroiditis. Years of tissue damage had unnecessarily occurred, and her thyroid may never fully recover. Had she received proper testing and treatment in the first place, she could have avoided this.

Additionally, even though she reported that gluten triggered swollen joints, no one had ever informed her about the severe consequences of eating gluten when you have an autoimmune disease. Small intermittent amounts of gluten fed her autoimmune thyroid disorder and caused further damage to her thyroid gland and joints. It's very likely she also had other autoimmune issues causing joint damage, which merited further testing.

The great news is that after beginning my Functional Ketogenic Gut Repair program, Suzy is healing well. Her symptoms are disappearing, her energy is returning, and her joints are no longer swollen and painful. She's changed her thinking and behaviors around food, is no longer using sugar to soothe emotional pain, is performing acts of self-love, and taking measures to own her power in her relationships.

THE SCIENCE
HOW YOUR IMMUNE SYSTEM WORKS

There are two main types of immune response: non-specific (cell-mediated) and specific (humoral). Immune-modulating cytokines (also known as interleukins and interferons) are the cells that help suppress or regulate immune responses. Some cytokines are secreted by cells known as T helper 1 (TH1)-type cells and others by T helper 2 (TH2)-type cells.

Non-specific immunity is produced by TH1 cells, and specific immunity by TH2 cells. These constitute the two arms of the immune system that often work together to fight infections. Non-specific immunity is the body's immediate response to infection: macrophages and natural killer T-cells attack microorganisms and abnormal cells at the place of infection inside cells. If they fail, then the specific system activates, producing antibodies by B-cells that help tag antigens, foreign invaders, and substances outside the cells for identification and destruction. Once tagged, they are easier for the TH1 system to identify and destroy.

If you have autoimmunity (as evidenced by significant levels of predictive antibodies, prior to symptoms) or autoimmune disease, some doctors recommend testing to determine if you are consistently TH1- or TH2-dominant, and to see how well your regulatory T-cells (called Treg cells for short) are functioning. They believe that knowing if you have a dominant aspect of your immune system—whether TH1 or TH2—can be helpful, although other doctors now argue that testing may not be accurate because our immune systems regularly morph in response to internal and external factors.

Ideally, the TH1 and TH2 systems should be dynamic and balanced, switching back and forth as needed. In chronic infection and autoimmunity, there is an imbalance between the two. Various subsets of Treg cells respond in times of infection and in allergic reaction, causing inflammation.

The vital importance of appropriate Treg cell suppression has been emphasized by Dr. Aristo Vojdani, who writes in the Cyrex Laboratories Clinical Application Guide to Array 5 that "inappropriate Treg cell frequency or functionality potentiates the pathogenesis of myriad diseases with ranging magnitudes of severity." This means that if your Treg cells aren't functioning properly, you are more likely to develop disease.

Many doctors and scientists have recently discovered that Treg cells are more beneficial in modulating immune function than previously thought. Various herbs and plant-derived polyphenols, such as turmeric and resveratrol, contain compounds that support "powerful immunoregulatory capacity via direct or indirect action on Treg cells," (Dr. Aristo Vojdani) and may relieve an inflammatory autoimmune attack or flare-up, thereby limiting collateral tissue damage.

In addition, probiotics induce production of Tr1 (Type 1 Treg) cells and Th3 cells. Lactobacillus casei propagates oral tolerance, which is the capacity of the immune system to recognize substances taken in through the digestive system and to weaken or suppress the immune response to them.

Autoimmunity and Your Gut

Let's look more closely at the structure of the digestive system and the process of digestion. The gastrointestinal tract starts at your teeth and extends to your anus.

The digestive process begins as you chew your food, a process known as mastication—an important, often overlooked phase of digestion. The simple act of chewing signals the entire gastrointestinal system to begin the complex process of digestion.

For example, chewing stimulates the pancreas to release digestive enzymes and bicarbonate into the lumen of the small intestine, while taste receptors in the mouth signal the lining of the stomach to produce hydrochloric acid, which is especially vital for digesting protein. Chewing breaks larger food particles into smaller ones, exposing much more surface area to digestive juices. If you don't chew well, large particles of food can remain undigested. Incomplete digestion encourages overgrowth of bad bacteria in the intestines, as the large particles stagnate in your gut and begin to putrefy, causing gas, bloating, constipation, and other digestive and immune problems.

A second essential function of chewing is to stimulate the saliva glands. Saliva helps clear away food in the mouth and lubricates the esophagus, making it easier to move the smaller food particles down. It helps wash away bacteria, which decreases plaque and thus reduces tooth decay. Saliva also contains important enzymes. Carbohydrate and fat digestion begin in the mouth with the secretion of salivary alpha-amylase and lingual lipase, which enable the stomach to further break them down so that the small intestine can absorb them.

Almost every patient I see shows signs of low digestive enzymes and hypochlorhydria (low stomach acid) because they don't chew their food sufficiently. I'm guilty myself. I used to scarf down my food because I was busy and hungry. I didn't realize how little I was actually chewing until I slowed down and began eating mindfully. This practice shifted my relationship with food and the act of nourishing my body. It also improved my digestive function.

Another benefit of thorough chewing is that you feel full faster, reducing the urge to overeat. You'll also enjoy the smell and taste of your food more when you take your time chewing. Some ancient yogic traditions actually taught students to chew each bite 50 times! A good gauge is if you can still identify which food is in your mouth. If you can detect any part of the food—stems, florets, leaves, and so on—then you haven't chewed enough. Bottom line: Food should be liquefied in your mouth.

And so, on to the intestines. Some 80 percent of your antibody-producing cells live in your GI tract. This makes it an immunological powerhouse, working either for or against you, day after day. Cultivating and supporting a healthy GI mucosal lining is imperative to your overall health and well-being. Be assured, whenever autoimmunity or autoimmune disease develops, the gut is in disarray. But what exactly is the connection between the gut and health?

Your intestines are lined with epithelial cells, which play two complementary roles: absorbing nutrients and forming a protective barrier that prevents incompletely digested food particles, microbes, and toxins from passing directly into the bloodstream.

Nutrients are absorbed through three structures:

- First, you absorb nutrients transcellularly—directly through the cells of the gut lining.
- Second, nutrients can pass paracellularly—between the cells. The pore-like structures known as tight junctions are small permeable openings located between the cells. The tight junctions seal the paracellular space between every cell in your gut lining.
- Third, nutrients can pass through the tiny crevices or webbing called *crypts* between the finger-like villi in the lining of the gut.

If any of these three methods of absorption are impaired, problems develop. When there's inflammation in the digestive tract, the tight junctions of the intestinal mucosa are compromised. This can occur through poor food choices; exposure to toxic chemicals, pathogenic bacteria, viruses, fungi, or parasites; eating non-organic foods; inadequate chewing; underproduction of stomach acid or digestive enzymes; stress; genetic factors; and dehydration, among other things.

The tight junctions are important because this is where nutrients are absorbed from the food you eat. If these pores in the lining of the GI tract remain open for too long, toxic byproducts and undigested food molecules are then absorbed into the bloodstream and transported to the liver, the chief detoxifying organ in your body. These toxic byproducts increase the toxic load on the liver, which struggles to metabolize them and keep you healthy. Eventually, the build-up causes symptoms of liver overload, such as headaches, brown blemishes on your skin known as liver spots, dark circles under the eyes, a yellowish tint to the whites of the eyes, gallstones, hormone imbalances, sluggish thyroid function, blood sugar problems, reduced metabolism leading to weight gain, and even cancer.

The toxins and food particles that leak into the bloodstream affect other systems throughout the body, aggravating any inflammation already present and triggering more inflammation, causing symptoms such as brain fog, neurotransmitter imbalances, food sensitivities, chemical sensitivities, and autoimmunity. Food particles are not meant to leak into the bloodstream. The body identifies these particles as foreign invaders, but the body isn't designed to be attacking food particles day in and day out.

If the tight junctions open too wide, or remain open too long, gut permeability is increased. Too many immune-signaling chemicals brought on by inflammation or stress can overstimulate the tight junctions and cause these pores to open too wide. This is considered to be a damaged mucosal barrier and leads to illness.

Breaches in the protective GI lining or boundary—known as gut hyper-permeability, or leaky gut—allow the entry of undigested antigens, toxins, and bacteria into the submucosa and directly into the bloodstream.

The immune system correctly identifies these substances as foreign invaders and launches a response. The steady barrage of such invaders eventually leads to immune overwhelm and confusion, which is the essence of autoimmunity (and allergies). The immune response feeds inflammation, and the cycle of intestinal permeability amplifies.

Symptoms associated with leaky gut include exhaustion, memory challenges, diarrhea, abdominal pain or bloating, chronic bacterial or yeast (candida) overgrowths, chronic sore throats and infections, fevers of unknown origin, difficulty concentrating, inflammation, swollen joints, headaches, allergies, and poor tolerance of exercise. As well, hyper-permeability is often an underlying factor in many conditions. These include skin disorders such as eczema and psoriasis; mood disorders such as depression, anxiety, and schizophrenia; irritable bowel syndrome; inflammatory bowel disease; chronic fatigue syndrome; attention deficit disorders; joint and collagen problems; multiple chemical sensitivities; compromised liver function; cystic fibrosis; ulcerative colitis; parasites; all autoimmune diseases; and cancer.

The Gut Microbiome: The Garden in Your Gut

The intestinal microbiota, also known as gut flora, is the community of microorganisms that resides in your intestines. We each have more bacterial cells in the intestines than we have human cells in the entire body. A human intestine is home to approximately 1,000 trillion microbes from 15,000 strains.[6] These microbes can add up to a weight of four to five pounds! The microbiota includes tens of trillions of microorganisms, with more than three million genes, constituting 150 times more genes than those found in your 46 human chromosomes. One-third of the gut microbiota is common to most people, while two-thirds is unique to you in a way that's similar to the uniqueness of your fingerprint or a snowflake.

Your intestinal microbiota is metabolically active and does not sit idle in your gut—it's either helping or hurting you. The microbiota facilitates immune and gastrointestinal development and maturation and modulation of the immune response. It has a tight relationship with you, its host, sensing stress in you and responding to it in many ways. In fact, a healthy intestinal microbiota is so important we should consider it another vital organ.

THE SCIENCE
BIOFILMS

Most microbes, both inside and outside the body, reside in a biofilm. Biofilms are protective mucilaginous coatings that encase colonies of bacteria and other microorganisms such as yeasts, fungi, and protozoa. Healthy biofilms and microbiota can prevent disease and support optimal health, while unhealthy ones create and sustain disease. Dental plaque is an example of a common biofilm. Also consider chronic infections, such as sinusitis, candida, or *Helicobacter pylori*, which often resist treatment due to their protective biofilms. Successful treatment first requires disruption of the biofilm in order to strip the pathogens of protection so they can be killed. Biofilms can be weakened with specific combinations of enzymes, herbs, probiotics, and pharmaceuticals.

Dr. Natalia Shulzhenko, assistant professor and physician in the Oregon State University Department of Biomedical Sciences, notes the importance of the gut microbiota in health and immunity: "The human gut plays a huge role in immune function. This is little appreciated by people who think its only role is digestion. The combined number of genes in the microbiota genome is 150 times larger than the person in which they reside. They do help us digest food, but they do a lot more than that."[7]

Commensal (symbiotic) bacteria, which do not harm the human host, communicate with the immune system in order to create adaptive lymphoid tissue and maintain healthy balanced intestines.[8] Shulzhenko's emerging theory of disease is a disruption in the "crosstalk" between the microbes in the human gut and other cells involved in the immune system and metabolic processes.

"In a healthy person, these microbes in the gut stimulate the immune system as needed," she says, "and it, in turn, talks back. [Unfortunately] there's an increasing disruption of these microbes from modern lifestyle, diet, overuse of antibiotics, and other issues. With that disruption, the conversation is breaking down."[9]

This breakdown leads to disease—especially autoimmune disease.

Another contributing factor to autoimmunity is lymphoid tissue. White blood cells, bone marrow, lymph nodes, leukocytes, thymus, and spleen are all lymphoid tissue and key players in immune function. And the GI tract possesses the largest mass of lymphoid tissue in the human body.[10] This gut-associated lymphoid tissue (GALT) is referred to as the "immune system" of the gastrointestinal tract, and GALT is made up of several types of lymphoid tissues that defend you from pathogens.

If you eat foods to which you have hidden sensitivities, or are exposed to toxins, bacteria, viruses, fungi, chemicals, or foreign substances, your GALT, the throne of your immune system, secretes antibodies to fight them. If you're prone to autoimmunity, or already have an autoimmune disease, this can create a cascade of inflammation and tissue damage. You may not notice until you have very uncomfortable symptoms and extensive tissue/organ damage. If your intestines are hyperpermeable (statistically likely), your immune system is not properly responding to food antigens, toxins, viruses, and bacteria. This can result in organ-specific diseases, including autoimmune diseases.

Celiac Disease

The poster child for the unhealthy gut is celiac disease, a digestive and autoimmune disorder that arises in response to the ingestion of wheat, other gluten-containing grains, or foods that cross-react with gluten, which can damage the lining of the small intestine and many other organs, causing a variety of symptoms. If the medical community had better testing when celiac disease was named, it would be considered a disease of the brain and other organs, more so than the gut because it more commonly impacts other organs than it does the small intestine.

Damage to the small intestine develops over time, beginning with inflammation and leading to atrophy of the finger-like, nutrient-absorbing villi. Gluten exposure can cause similar damage to occur in other organs and glands, such as the thyroid, until enough tissue damage has occurred that a formal diagnosis can be made.

But even if you haven't been diagnosed with celiac disease, ulcerative colitis, or IBD, your gut is likely to be in need of repair. Just look at what and how you've been eating. A reliable recipe for gut damage includes a diet of foods that are processed, microwaved, genetically modified, laden with pesticides and preservatives (non-organics), and loaded with carbs. Even a strictly raw or vegan diet can be problematic if the food is eaten while rushed, in the car, and consumed with popular drinks like coffee and soda rather than pure spring water. Other ingredients in the recipe for gut damage are stress, trauma, unresolved emotional struggles, environmental toxins, chronic dehydration, lack of adequate and deep sleep, lack of proper exercise, thyroid disorders (even if they are being treated with medication), and pharmaceutical drugs, such as antibiotics, antihistamines, anti-depressants, and beta blockers.

To the degree that any of these patterns occur in your history, you will have gut damage and need to restore homeostasis to your gastrointestinal system through gut repair and reflorination (re-establishing healthy intestinal bacteria).

Your Other Brain: The Enteric Nervous System

The enteric nervous system (ENS) was first described in 1921 by John Newport Langley, professor of physiology at Cambridge University in Britain. He believed it was one of three parts of the autonomic nervous system, which controls involuntary actions, such as heartbeat, blood pressure, and breathing. His work was mostly forgotten until Dr. Michael D. Gershon, author of *The Second Brain*, reintroduced the concept, suggesting that the gut both makes and uses some of the same neurotransmitters as the brain. His work was widely ridiculed, but now we have enough scientific evidence to prove its validity.

The brain and the gut—the central and enteric nervous systems—are deeply connected, but perhaps not in the ways you may have guessed. They each have their own control centers and can function separately. Please reread that last sentence and contemplate that for just a moment. The ENS is the supervisor of all digestive function, from the esophagus to the stomach, small intestine, and colon. This nearly self-contained second brain implements sophisticated neural circuitry, neurotransmitters, and proteins to get the job done, very much like the brain encased in your skull.

The ENS does all of this with very little help from the central nervous system (CNS). The ENS contains more than a hundred million nerve cells, which is roughly equal to the number of nerve cells in your spinal cord. If you consider the nerve cells in the other parts of your digestive system, such as your esophagus and stomach, it adds up to even more.

We know that the brain and the central nervous system can affect bowel motility, ion transport associated with secretion and absorption, and gastrointestinal blood flow. We also know that if the thin strand of a few thousand nerve fibers running from the brain to the one hundred million nerve cells in the small intestine were severed, the ENS would continue to function efficiently on its own. This means you would still be able to digest, absorb, and eliminate without your brain or central nervous system.

And here's something equally amazing. Peristaltic reflex refers to the wave-like muscular contractions of your digestive tract as it moves waste through the large intestine and out. The peristaltic reflex is initiated when the pressure inside the intestines (intraluminal pressure) increases, stimulating enterochromaffin cells to release serotonin, which further stimulates vagal and enteric afferent nerve fibers.

This may sound complex, and it is. But here's the point: Your gut makes serotonin, the neurotransmitter that improves your mood and makes your outlook on life stay sunny. So when I say a healthy gut means a happier life, you know I'm not kidding around! Before I detail my therapeutic, functional ketogenic gut repair plan, I'd like to share a few important missing pieces to the conventional view of nutrition, stress, your body, and gut damage.

Chapter 2

A Crucial Factor and Fresh View of Your Body

We've explored the more "conventional" scientific aspects of your gut and immune function but there is more. The concepts in this chapter are likely new and perhaps even shocking, so take your time as I introduce you to a completely new way of viewing your body and life. These perspectives back up a truly functional ketogenic gut repair program because they go beyond just a diet and embody a more balanced way of being.

It goes without saying that food is of central importance when it comes to healing your gut and re-establishing balance in your life, but it's not the only factor; there are several critical considerations to bring healing back into your life that go beyond food. These include unpacking the "body burden" you've accumulated from birth onward, unraveling and rethinking your relationship with stress, and attending to the needs of your "emotional gut."

The term "body burden" refers to the accumulation of toxins, heavy metals, pesticides, chemicals, pharmaceuticals, air and water pollution, beauty care chemicals, food preservatives, and flavor enhancers in your physical body. Your body can also become burdened with unresolved emotions from trauma, abuse, neglect, accidents, and environmental catastrophes. Diving deeply into body burden is outside the scope of this book, so please look for upcoming books that explore this fascinating topic.

Stress: The Silent Killer

Homeostasis is the state where your internal physiology, emotions, and psychology remain stable despite what's going on in the external world. It is our natural state. Stress occurs when anything seriously threatens homeostasis. Once this delicate balance is disturbed, it impacts our mood, informs our actions, and controls both our sense of well-being and our health.

Stress and trauma are prolific in our culture. The nature of the stress, your perception of it, its duration/persistence, the amount of stress or number of stressful events or situations, plus your genetics and constitution determine how stress affects you. As you age, the long-term effects of stress accumulate, and every aspect of your physical body and psyche is affected.

The number of people experiencing truly traumatic events is high in the West, with estimates ranging from 40 to 70 percent. In my practice, almost every woman I've ever seen has experienced some level of trauma and violence in her life, usually sexual, which often leads to health issues.

Metabolic Syndrome—the name for a group of risk factors that increase a person's risk for heart disease, diabetes, and stroke—is strongly influenced by stress. Symptoms include weight gain, especially around the middle, and dyslipidemia (elevated cholesterol or triglycerides, or both), often accompanied by low HDL (high density lipoprotein).

Stress from relationships and overall perceived stress are associated with weight gain, especially among women. Stressed mothers produce fewer antibodies and are therefore unable to provide the barrier against disease to their infants. Stress has been shown to elevate blood pressure (BP). A study of 7,066 male participants with a high level of general stress revealed that they had more than twice the risk of developing Type 2 diabetes during the 10-year follow-up.

Exposure to intense and chronic stressors during developmental years, such as violence, abuse, marital conflict, and divorce, has "long-lasting neurobiological effects and puts one at increased risk for anxiety and mood disorders, aggressive dyscontrol problems, hypo-immune dysfunction, medical morbidity, structural changes in the CNS, and early death."

Stress can also drive self-destructive bad habits, such as smoking, overeating, sugar addiction, and other kinds of substance abuse. It leads to poor sleep and sometimes even accidents that could have been avoided.

Chronic stress also releases hormones that suppress the immune system by affecting pro-inflammatory cytokines. As a result, stress can trigger harmful autoimmune responses. A stress response that is chronically activated and dysregulated fuels autoimmune inflammation and tissue destruction. In healthy individuals, cortisol would be produced to stop the inflammation, but in people with autoimmunity this is not the case, and the cycle of pro-inflammatory cytokine production continues indefinitely.

Fortunately, there are many psychosocial interventions available. Cognitive behavioral therapy (CBT) is effective, as is cognitive-behavioral stress management (CBSM), rapid eye movement techniques like EMDR, psychotherapy, MDMA-facilitated psychotherapy, meditation, and advanced techniques creating heart/brain coherence developed by the HeartMath Institute of California. I've also seen incredible healing through advanced somato-emotional release, homeopathy, NADA ear acupuncture protocol, full body acupuncture, family constellation work, and the LifeLine Technique®, all of which can be used in various combinations to help you regain homeostasis, emotional freedom, and deep peace.

Seeking help is an act of self-love. I fully believe in the team approach, working with other healthcare providers, trauma specialists, and psychotherapists—whatever it takes—to holistically support deep healing on all levels.

The Body as a Garden versus Machine

This book would be incomplete without addressing the emotional and spiritual components of your gastrointestinal health. First, let me share an ancient concept that is likely new to you and has informed a great deal of my understanding of how emotions impact your body.

In Traditional Chinese Medicine (TCM), the human body is viewed as a garden, representing a microcosm of the surrounding universe. In this view, the plants themselves, the soil, the microbiome and soil nutrients, minerals, insects, birds, sun, rain, and temperature are metaphors for your body's physiological systems—your organs, glands, tissues, blood, bones, ligaments, muscles, and cells. Like a garden, where all the elements work together to create a healthy, bountiful crop of food, the systems in your body synergistically work together to create health and physical well-being.

The plants in the garden are grown and harvested during their correct season. The gardener (the Doctor of Asian Medicine) knows this schedule and honors it. The gardener/practitioner works in harmony with the plants and surrounding environment to ensure the plants are healthy and strong. The seedlings and plants are sown and tended according to their individual needs—some plants need less water than others; some need more sun or more shade. The gardener/practitioner weeds out invasive, poisonous plants, often planting companion plants that strengthen their neighbors. They cultivate the soil (soul) so that the plants can grow and produce in abundance (as you produce in your job, relationships, achieving goals, making money, and so on).

The entire gardening process is a synergistic dance between all the elements of the garden and the gardener, who assists the garden in maintaining its balance, growth, and optimum performance.

Contrast this view with the Western medical view of the body as a machine and the doctor as mechanic. The mechanic views the machine as comprised of many uniform and standardized parts. Standardization makes replacing the parts simple. For example, when a group of people are given the same lab test, such as TSH for the thyroid, they receive their diagnosis based on the limitations of that test and receive the same treatment. No attention is paid to their individuality or the causes of any imbalance or irregularity. This is known as the Standard of Care in Western medicine.

In actuality, TSH is a marker of pituitary health as much as thyroid function. And there are 10 markers of thyroid health to both read and understand in order to find the root issue in thyroid conditions that the TSH doesn't address. But the mechanic isn't interested in this information because it isn't standardized.

In the mechanic's view, the body is divided into systems similar to mechanical processes. For example, the electrical system of your car may be seen as your central nervous system. The cardiovascular system that pumps oxygenated blood through your body is like the engine and fuel system of a car. In this view, the door is separate from the gas gauge, and either can be replaced. Which is why surgical intervention is so popular in Western medicine.

Unlike the gardener, who knows that every individual aspect of the garden affects the whole, the mechanic believes that individual parts of your machine, such as the engine, can be removed, repaired, or replaced without any impact on the other parts of your machine. The fuel line can be flushed without any impact on the air conditioner. And the mechanic/doctor replaces the broken part or uses duct tape and glue (pharmaceuticals) to keep things patched together without ever acknowledging the root cause of the mechanical issue or the other things the problem might be affecting.

But think about this: Just imagine your oil light comes on in your car, and instead of adding oil to the engine, you slap a piece of tape over the light and keep driving. What happens? Your engine eventually overheats, seizes, and dies. Symptoms in your body are like the oil light coming on in your car. The symptoms are information telling you something needs to be corrected. Taking drugs or submitting to invasive procedures that don't identify and treat the root cause of the symptoms (the oil light) is you covering up the warning light.

This stark contrast between the body as a garden and the body as machine is one of the many reasons that acupuncture and other holistic modalities are becoming so popular today. Yes, I began my personal healing and professional medical journey within the Western medicine paradigm, and I believe it has its place. But its philosophy of healing is fundamentally out of alignment with how life functions.

Honoring the Emotional Gut (Your Gut Has Feelings, Too!)

Even Western science is beginning to see the connection between emotions and health. For example, people who get angry when their self-esteem is threatened exhibit increases in the stress hormone cortisol. Negative emotions in general have been found to potentially play a role in developing coronary heart disease (CHD).

The heart, recognized in many cultures as the seat of love and compassion, is undoubtedly impacted by all emotions. Have you ever felt "heart-broken," experienced "heart-ache," or felt a "hole in your heart"? Situations and circumstances that elicit such heart-felt sensations impact more than your emotional state; they impact your entire physiology.

In the TCM view, organs house energy and vitality and when influenced by negative emotions, can become unbalanced, developing into symptoms or an illness. And just as there are companion plants in a garden, the organs of the human body are paired as well. For example, the large intestine is a paired organ with the lungs and the small intestine is paired with the heart. Just like with companion plants, this means they work together energetically and impact the health or imbalance of each other. The lungs can store grief, sadness, and regret. The intestines can become inflamed with emotions such as suppressed sadness, anger, frustration, craving, and fear.

In the Asian medical model, the heart pairs with the mind and is responsible for cognitive activities, memory, emotions, and sleep. It also pairs with the small intestines. Although there isn't a strong connection between the heart and small intestines physiologically, there certainly is emotionally and mentally. In Western physiology, we know the small intestines absorb nutrients. However, in TCM, the small intestines are understood to absorb much more, including emotions, beliefs, stress, anxiety, trauma, and reactive patterns from our family of origin, such as patterns of abuse, neglect, anger, poor boundaries, codependency, addiction, and lack of self-love. All of these things directly impact how the small intestines function physically, and therefore gut health.

As you struggle with loss, grief, fear, anger, trauma or regret, remember that your body must also process these emotions and your biological needs change when you are under stress. Fully feeling your emotions is an important step to healing.

Body Memory

There are dozens and dozens of healing modalities to address stress, trauma, and unresolved emotions that are literally stuck in your tissues. I briefly introduce a few so you can begin your own exploration.

John Upledger, a founding father of craniosacral therapy and the Upledger Institute, and author of *Your Inner Physician*, taught that every experience and every emotion is stored in the body and that our cells remember past events and distress. He developed Dr. William Sutherland's initial form of craniosacral therapy—a powerful yet gentle treatment that works with the natural, self-correcting mechanism of the body to detect and release restrictions in mobility and enhance function.

The work of Dr. Darren Weissman, creator of the Lifeline Technique® and author of *Unlocking the Secret Code of Your Mind*, also addresses the subconscious patterns, beliefs, and memories stored in our bodies. He asserts that "the body speaks the mind," and I agree. As an example, consider constipation—being impacted with fecal matter. What are you holding onto? What are you struggling to maintain control over? Now, consider diarrhea. What are you not able to assimilate in your life? What is too painful for you to handle? Do you lack boundaries? Do your emotions spill out in inappropriate ways? Are you codependent? Do you suppress your emotions so your body must find other ways of releasing? These are just a few of the questions to be investigated when honoring the body–mind–spirit connection and gut health.

There are dozens of other wonderfully effective techniques for resolving past trauma. The work of Dr. Joe Dispenza, author of *Breaking The Habit of Being Yourself*, is filled with easy-to-understand science as well as self-help meditations to help people change their brain wave patterns, awaken the pineal gland, and shift their biological processes. I've personally received incredible benefit from working with him.

Other methods include eye movement desensitization and repro-cessing (EMDR), EFT (Emotional Freedom Technique), Bruno Chikly's brain techniques, acupuncture, Holotropic Breathwork™, psychosomatic sessions of body and face reading with specific alignment corrections, flower essences, many forms of movement therapy, dolphin and equine-assisted or interspecies-facilitated therapy, sound therapy, homeopathy, shamanic soul retrieval, kambo, MDMA-facilitated psychotherapy, and plant medicines, to name just a few of my favorites.

I know some (or all) of this may sound foreign to you and far out. But all of these modalities work. As a holistic therapist and human being who has taken her own healing journey, I want to give you everything I've got. I want to connect all the dots for you when it comes to the amazing, intricate dance between your mind, your body, your spirit and all the possible pathways you can take towards experiencing greater resilience, harmony, happiness, and health. Your gut health depends on a comprehensive approach to your well-being. I heartily recommend finding the healthcare professionals and approaches that resonate with you and embarking on your own exploration.

Chapter 3

Dietary Evolution and the Functional Ketogenic Approach

Let's explore our human evolution and how my functional ketogenic approach fits. The Paleolithic era, also called the Stone Age, spans a period from about 2.6 million years ago to 10,000 years ago. Agriculture began during the Neolithic period (roughly 10,000 to 2,000 B.C.) after the last glacial ice receded. Archaeological evidence establishes this as the time that the nomadic lifestyle of humans was replaced by the first settlements in villages, the cultivation of crops, and the establishment of animal husbandry. Evidence of the first use of agriculture has been found in the area known as the Fertile Crescent (now Iraq, Syria and adjoining region).

During the Paleolithic era, humans and their immediate ancestors had the same fundamental physiology as you and I have today. And you know how they ate? They hunted and gathered, feeding on wild game meat, animal fats, and wild plants, with minimal intake of fruits such as berries. They also consumed wild grasses and their seeds. But those were not so attractive because of the processing needed to make them edible and because the caloric rewards were limited.

Looking back some 150,000 generations, the bones and teeth of our ancestors confirm that we come from a long line of hunter gatherers. Their tools also exhibit evidence of an omnivorous diet.

Anthropologists have found animal bones with teeth marks overlain by tool cut marks, telling the story of a carnivore kill followed by human scavenging. Conversely, other bones show cut marks followed by sharp teeth marks, suggesting an initial kill by a human with a weapon, followed by an animal scavenger. These findings were proven through dietary isotopic composition and by the lack of grass-consumption scratch marks on their teeth, meaning they were meat eaters.

Compared to other primates, human brains are proportionally twice as large, while our digestive tracts are 60 percent smaller. Which means we require nutrient-dense food. Among primates, the vegetarian gorilla has proportionally the smallest brain and largest digestive system—the polar opposites of humans. Some vegetarians argue that gorillas—fueled by their vegetarian diet—are big and strong, so we can be as well. However, gorillas have a vital advantage that we humans lack: fermentative bacteria in their guts necessary for digesting cellulose.[11] The "expensive tissue hypothesis," coined by anthropologists Leslie Aiello and Peter Wheeler, argues that the Australopithecine brain grew to *Homo sapiens* proportions because meat consumption allowed our digestive systems to shrink, which freed up energy for our brains to grow.[12]

Evolution works slowly, and not enough time has elapsed since the advent of agriculture—a mere 10,000 years—for our species' digestive system to adapt to a vegetarian lifestyle. Which is sad news for vegetarians and vegans.

If you have further doubts about how poorly our digestive systems are geared for vegetarianism, I strongly encourage you to read *Primal Body, Primal Mind: Beyond the Paleo Diet for Total Health and a Longer Life* by Nora T. Gedgaudas. In this book, she brilliantly documents the evolution of our hominid ancestors up to the present era, explaining why they ate as they did, how diets changed with the rise of agriculture, and why that has been so ruinous to our health. She provides the science to prove her case and gives specific recommendations on how we can remedy those problems and thrive.

And if evolution hasn't yet prepared us for a simple vegetarian diet, it most assuredly hasn't prepared our bodies to handle the onslaught of carbohydrates and dairy, processed, de-natured, sugar-laden, artificial-ingredient-saturated, trans fat-filled food we've grown accustomed to eating in the last 50 years.

So, what are we to do?

The healthy solution—simple in concept, yet counter to all of our mis-informed cultural conditioning—is the functional ketogenic gut repair plan.

Chapter 4

Ketogenic Benefits versus Paleo and Primal

The ketogenic-type diet was originally developed as a medical intervention and alternative to prolonged fasting for children with epilepsy in the 1920s and 1930s. Standard ketogenic foods include: meats, fatty fish, eggs, butter, cream, cheese, non-starch or low-carb vegetables, healthy oils, avocados, nuts, and seeds. Ninety percent dark chocolate is also allowed.

However, this book is written for people ready to take a healing journey toward gut repair. My Functional Ketogenic Gut Repair Plan excludes all dairy, eggs, soy, nuts and seeds, and chocolate for the first two to four months, as well as any other gut-damaging and inflammatory foods. (Please see chapter "Food: The Foundation of Keto Gut Repair" for details.) But that doesn't mean my program can't be modified after the healing process is complete and used as a healthy, long-term functional ketogenic nutritional plan that, with modifications for individual needs and lifestyles, is excellent for athletes and any other health-conscious human being.

Mainstream Ketogenic Diets

Standard Ketogenic Diet (SKD): This is a very low-carb, moderate-protein, high-fat diet. It typically contains 75 percent fat, 20 percent protein, and only 5 percent carbs. These are the therapeutic food ratios that I'm advocating with a gut repair plan.

High-Protein Ketogenic Diet (HPKD): This is similar to a standard ketogenic diet but includes more protein. The ratio is often 60 percent fat,

35 percent protein, and 5 percent carbs. This isn't the most ideal because people don't require this much protein; however, it can work for some athletes, especially weightlifters.

Cyclical Ketogenic Diet (CKD): This diet involves periods of higher-carb refeeds, such as five ketogenic days followed by two high-carb days. This allows the glycogen storage in the muscles to be refueled. This is not something I recommend for gut repair, but it can work for some people after healing is complete. It can be stressful for your body to change how it is metabolizing, and it may take longer than a week to really get into ketosis, so you don't necessarily receive the long-term benefits. This is often used for people who are really pushing their bodies to the limits of athletic performance.

Targeted Ketogenic Diet (TKD): This diet allows you to add carbs around workouts. In my opinion, this defeats the whole purpose of gaining benefit from the ketogenic diet. Athletes receive huge benefit, and taking in carbs around a workout can rob them of many ketogenic perks. It's mostly used with beginner and intermediate body builders and endurance athletes who may be hitting a wall during their intense training. It's not meant to be therapeutic.

Benefits of a Ketogenic Diet

Aside from the fact that you'll feel better overall and live a happier, longer life, there are many specific health benefits to a ketogenic diet along with the therapeutic differences and importance of a functional ketogenic gut repair program.

Uncontrolled epilepsy, or intractable epileptic seizures, is the first disorder that the ketogenic diet was proven to greatly diminish and even cure, because of how the brain functions more optimally on ketones than glucose alone. One study had a three- to six-year follow-up of 150 children with difficult-to-control seizures. Not only were these seizures controlled but the diet allowed the decrease or discontinuation of medication. The ketogenic diet is more effective than the newer anticonvulsant medications.

In 1924, more children with epilepsy were studied and pediatric physician Dr. M. G. Peterman found that cognitive abilities increased and mood stabilized, leading to behavioral improvements in children who followed the ketogenic diet. Mental development was normal to exceptional, seizures ceased and the children slept better.

There is research pointing to the therapeutic benefits of a ketogenic diet for people with malignant brain tumors. KetoCal®, a nutritionally complete, ketogenically balanced medical food, was used in a study. (**Note:** This product is not gut repair-friendly because it contains whey and milk, as well as artificial flavors, soy, and corn starch). In the ketogenic/restricted calorie group, researchers noted a decrease in the intracerebral growth of the CT-2A and U87-MG tumors by about 65 percent and 35 percent, respectively. The patients also had significantly enhanced health and survival relative to that of the control groups receiving the standard low-fat/high-carbohydrate diet. They found that these brain tumors have reduced ability to metabolize ketone bodies for energy, so they shrank due to lack of food. While the tumors lacked food, the rest of the body did not.[13]

A very low-carbohydrate diet (VLCD), 20 grams/day, has been shown to significantly improve moderate to severe symptoms, such as abdominal pain, stool habits like frequency and consistency (research concluded a significant decrease in stool frequency as well as improvement in stool consistency), and quality of life in people suffering from irritable bowel syndrome (IBS) with a predominance of diarrhea (IBS-D). Another finding of the study was that overweight and obese individuals initiating a VLCD had a profound clinical response in their IBS-D symptoms.[14]

In fact, carbohydrates are well known to exacerbate symptoms of IBS. Most people with IBS have carbohydrate fermentation problems in their gut. This impacts immune function and furthers dysbiosis (imbalance of bad and good gut microbes), leading to lifelong symptoms and stress that are completely avoidable.

In sum, a ketogenic diet has innumerable benefits for your body and mind. Here are a few more scientifically proven effects:

BENEFITS OF KETOGENIC DIET

- Increases glutathione production, which means anti-aging, natural detoxification, and brain health
- Increases BDBF gene expression
- Increases mitochondria concentration, which means more energy
- Stimulates hematopoietic stem cells
- Reduces inflammatory molecules (leptin, IFNy, IL-6, IL- IB)
- Reduces oxidative stress at the mitochondria

The ketogenic diet provides a solid foundation for gut repair, although a few refinements are needed before it becomes optimal. An unmodified ketogenic diet still contains common high-allergen foods, notably eggs, dairy, nightshades, and nuts. But the functional ketogenic gut repair plan detailed in this book will give you powerful gut-healing tools and support.

Paleo and Primal

When it comes to food and diets, emotions can run hot over the details. Everybody has an opinion! If you're at all familiar with the Paleo and Primal diets, you already know there are similarities and differences between them and the ketogenic approach. To avoid any confusion, I thought it best to include a brief chapter covering them.

The Paleo diet has evolved over the years since Loren Cordain popularized the caveman diet in his 2002 book, *The Paleo Diet*. Cordain's eating formula includes nuts and seeds, lean meats, fish, eggs in moderation, roots, vegetables, wild berries, no sugar, no added salt, no alcohol, no coffee, no grains, no soy, no dairy, an avoidance of processed foods, but shockingly, artificial sweeteners are allowed (many people who follow a Paleo diet don't use them.)

One problem with this particular approach from the ketogenic standpoint is the lack of saturated fats. Our ancestors used the entire carcass of the animal they killed. The prized parts were the organ meats, bone marrow, and fatty deposits. As we've seen, humans need fat. Our brains are made up of mostly cholesterol, and fats play an important role in healthy neurological functioning. Without healthy saturated fats like coconut oil, we're left with processed polyunsaturated products. This certainly isn't what the human body was designed to solely utilize for brain health.

Followers of the Primal diet concur. The Primal diet (which attracted the world's attention around 2010 with the publication of triathlete and Ironman competitor Mark Sisson's first publication, *The Primal Blueprint Cookbook*), recognizes saturated fats as a neutral, stable source of fat, important for energy, neurological function, hormone manufacture, and cellular structure. As well, while the Primal diet acknowledges that dairy can be problematic, it maintains that full-fat dairy (preferably raw) from pasture-raised animals is a healthy source of fat, protein, and calcium.

The Primal diet also includes coffee (Paleo does not). The Primal diet is also more lenient as far as legumes and fermented soy products are concerned.

Here's a quick summary of the similarities between Paleo and Primal lifestyles:

- Both avoid grains
- Both eliminate gluten
- Both do away with corn
- Both avoid high-fructose corn syrup
- Both avoid other sugars
- Both eliminate processed foods
- Both include tons of veggies
- Both include lots of protein
- Both include regular exercise

There are also lifestyle differences between Paleo and Primal. Paleo focuses on diet over exercise, while Primal is a more holistic approach, including more exercise and nutrition. Primal encourages you to move your body, use your brain, get plenty of sleep, lift heavy things, avoid toxins, avoid trauma, sprint occasionally, get sunlight daily, and play.

Paleo and Primal Concerns

Currently in North America and most of the civilized world, we're not hunting and gathering. We're not living in the wild. We're not expending large amounts of energy to track, kill, and prepare wild game. Our nutritional needs are different from our Paleolithic ancestors'.

Some scientists argue that 10,000 years of evolution is plenty of time to adapt to the inclusion of dairy, grains, and legumes; however, the high rates of lactose intolerance, gluten sensitivity disorders, gastrointestinal disorders, and immune dysfunction, including cancer (even in young children), are glaring pieces of evidence to the contrary. As well, domesticated plants and animals have a vastly different nutritional profile than they did in the Paleolithic era. Also, there were no such plants as broccoli, cauliflower, or kale, all of which are full of highly beneficial nutrients.

Our lifestyle, genetics, individual nutritional needs, and health status inform what, how, and when we should eat. There is no one size fits all. For example, when I have a heavy workout, I need more calorie-dense foods. I'm currently using my Functional Ketogenic Gut Repair Program to help heal my gut, so increasing healthy fat intake is essential, especially when I'm working out. Not everyone will need the same thing. I have a dear friend who has a faster metabolism. When he works out, he needs almost three times as much food, even on my program, in order to stay feeling healthy and strong. He remains muscular, lean, and energized, even with twice as many meals as I need. Your needs are likely different.

Chapter 5

The Functional Ketogenic Gut Repair Basics

First off, please note that when I talk about diet I'm not talking about the modern concept of the word—a fad formula of eating you painfully embrace for a few weeks in order to lose weight on some crash program. The Functional Ketogenic Gut Repair Program is the exact opposite of a fad diet. It might be better and more accurate to call it the Functional Ketogenic Lifestyle, because this is about making an overall nutritional, lifestyle, and attitudinal change about your food and health.

Secondly, please note that *ketosis* is not the same thing as *keto-acidosis*. Sometimes people misunderstand and confuse these two terms. Ketoacidosis is a dangerous metabolic state that can even be fatal, most often occurring in untreated Type 1 (insulin-dependent) diabetics. There is some debate as to whether a ketogenic diet is healthy for people with any type of diabetes. The literature points to positive benefits in preventing, halting, and even reversing diabetes symptoms by lowering blood glucose and hemoglobin A1c levels. This is especially effective for Type 2 (non-insulin-dependent, that is, "adult onset") diabetes, and is effective in Type 1 diabetes with the guidance of a knowledgeable healthcare practitioner. It's also necessary to support the liver and immune function because many people with diabetes have unidentified immune dysfunction and fatty liver disease from insulin resistance.

I recently had a patient on two different diabetic medications. She was clinically obese (at least 95 lbs overweight), diagnosed with Hashimoto's thyroiditis, and struggling. After several weeks of exploring her inner world around food addiction and fat tissue as protection, she began my Functional Ketogenic Gut Repair Program.

In the first week, she dropped from five pills of Metformin to three, then two; she lost 7 lbs; and her energy rose while her blood sugar dropped. She didn't have one sugar craving! We worked with her doctor in the following weeks to safely reduce her medications even more. By week six, she was completely free of all medication, approved by her physician. She was reaching her goal of healing and curing her symptoms of Type II Diabetes, losing weight, and halting the autoimmune thyroid condition. If she can do it, so can you.

Ketosis is the metabolic state in which the body relies primarily on fats rather than carbohydrates for fuel. It's the natural (and desirable) state to evoke, because over millions of years we've evolved to store fat when food is abundant and to burn fat when food is scarce. This is the essential formula for a true ketogenic-type nutritional plan. After all, most of us aren't going without food for extended periods as our ancestors once did. And Paleo diets that feature high-carbohydrate foods, such as starchy root vegetables that appeal to sugar/carb addicts, fail to deliver the metabolic benefits of a high-fat, low-carbohydrate, true ketogenic-type diet.

Unlike other diets, the Functional Ketogenic Gut Repair Program:

- is high in healthy fat—approximately 60–75 percent of calories (gasp!);
- is adequate in protein (2–4 oz/60–120 g twice per day, depending on your weight and exercise, or 20 percent of calories);
- is low in carbohydrates (1 oz/30 g or less per day, or 5 percent of calories);
- is free of grain-based and starchy vegetable carbs;
- is high in a wide variety of vegetables;
- focuses on gut repair (unlike any other ketogenic type diet, which include gut-damaging foods like dairy and eggs);
- empowers you with the info you need to have appropriate functional testing;
- addresses stress, hydration, exercise, and sleep (see Part III);
- acknowledges the emotional aspects of the gut, offering guided introspective exercises (see Part III).

Part II

Fun Facts about Food as Your Medicine

The other major TCM philosophy that changed my life is the view of food as medicine. TCM practitioners honor the flavors, seasons, colors, temperature, and energetics of food, using them to work with imbalances in the body, mind, and spirit. It is understood that foods enter specific channels of energy called meridians and work with the organ associated with that meridian. Foods and herbs work in conjunction with acupuncture and other Asian medical techniques to support the entire system to remember balance and adaptability.

Eating with the seasons is another part of using food as medicine. Asian medicine honors not only the energetics of food and their nutrients but also when and how that food was grown, harvested, stored, and prepared. This comprehensive approach to nutrition incorporates the scientific measurements of nutrients as well as the energetic properties and lifestyle components. The next step of viewing food as medicine is working with how that food is then prepared and consumed. Denatured food is food that has been robbed of its nutrients or altered to retain less nutritional value. Processing and microwaving food are two examples of ways in which food is denatured.

My approach to using food as medicine works to raise your awareness while offering you new tools to implement in your current food and life practices. In the food section of this book I list the energetics of the foods used in each recipe.

I hope you find the added information and "flavor" of TCM beneficial in your healing journey. I would like to see you become an informed health consumer. I believe it is far healthier and more affordable for someone to get regular acupuncture than to take a dozen prescription drugs trying to alleviate symptoms and then have to deal with the consequences.

Chapter 6

Busting the Myths about Carbs and Fat

We need a steady source of fuel for our bodies to run efficiently. Simple carbohydrates (sugars, starches, and grains) burn quickly and don't last. They also cause spikes in insulin. All carbohydrates are converted into glucose, and the irregular spikes in insulin and blood sugar stress the body. By contrast, complex carbohydrates from vegetables and certain fruit sources are metabolized more efficiently and smoothly by the body. (I highly recommend two books by Stephen D. Phinney and Jeff S. Volek: *The Art and Science of Low Carbohydrate Living* and *The Art and Science of Low Carbohydrate Performance*.)

The body can only store 2,000 kilocalories of carbohydrates as glycogen in your muscles. Once consumed, it's gone until the metabolic pantry can be restocked. When glycogen stores are consumed, you experience what many athletes refer to as "bonking"—a sudden collapse of energy. If you get cranky or tired when you miss a meal, now you know why. You've "bonked." Conversely, fat cells have a large capacity for storage, and fat contains nine kilocalories per gram. The body can thus store and use more than 40,000 kilocalories as fat![15]

You know you can get a burst of energy from carbohydrates—and you also have felt that it doesn't last. During prolonged exercise, when the body's carbohydrates stored as glycogen are being depleted, there is increasing dependence on the liver to maintain blood glucose levels. This is not just to provide the exercising muscles with glucose but also to support other normal body functions, particularly those of the central nervous system.[16]

Vigorous exercise depletes glycogen reserves in a few hours. Diets with an emphasis on carbohydrates bias the metabolism toward carbs, while inhibiting fat metabolism and utilization.[17] But when the metabolic system is tuned to primarily burn fat, there are several days' worth of fuel available.[18] Consider our Neanderthal ancestors. If a hunter's only hope of eating in the coming months is to track a herd of woolly mammoths for days with no snacks available, would he choose a source of long-lasting energy or a source that would only give him short spurts? And if a saber-toothed tiger were chasing him, wouldn't he prefer to outrun it without bonking?

As a biology major and pre-med student, I was taught that the brain runs on glucose. But guess what? In actual fact, the brain runs as much as 25 percent better on *fat,* in the form of ketones! There are only a few parts of your brain that need glucose, and this can be converted from ketones. Too much glucose can, in fact, be damaging to the brain. The journal *Medical Hypothesis* published an interesting article outlining that HC (high-carbohydrate) foods are the primary cause of Alzheimer's disease (AD). There are two mechanisms by which this occurs. First is the inhibition of membrane proteins such as glucose transporters and the amyloid precursor protein, which occurs because of disturbances in lipid metabolism in the central nervous system. Second is damage to cerebral neurons by prolonged and increased insulin signaling. This naturally points to nutritional changes, primarily carbohydrate decreases or restriction, while increasing essential fatty acids (EFA), as a feasible prevention strategy.[19] That's correct: diet can prevent and treat Alzheimer's disease.

Your brain is 60 percent saturated fat, and 25 percent of the brain consists of cholesterol. A ketogenic diet includes lots of fat—including healthy *saturated* fat—in the form of organic, unrefined coconut oil and duck and lamb fat. Trust me, your brain, hair, skin, nails, immune system, and heart will thank you! Coconut contains lauric acid, which has strong antiviral and antifungal properties and is also an immune system builder. Unsaturated fats such as olive oil lower total blood cholesterol, "bad" LDL cholesterol, and triglycerides while at the same time supporting levels of "good" HDL cholesterol, which plays a protective role in the body.

Serotonin receptors in the brain also need cholesterol, because it counters depression.[20] In *The Vegetarian Myth,* author Lierre Keith cites an interesting double-blind study done by a British researcher on a psychologically healthy group of people who were not under any stress. All meals eaten during the study were supplied by the researchers. One group's diet was 41 percent fat-based and the other contained only 25 percent fat. After a period of time, the researchers switched the groups, so the low-fat dieters ate the high-fat diet, and vice versa.

Each volunteer in the study underwent thorough psychological testing before and after each trial. The results? While ratings of anger-hostility slightly declined during the high-fat diet period, they significantly increased during the low-fat, high-carbohydrate diet period. Similarly, ratings of depression declined slightly during the high-fat period but increased during the low-fat period. Levels of anxiety declined during the high-fat period but did not change during the four weeks of low-fat eating.[21]

Ketogenic diets also increase the production of BDNF (brain-derived neurotrophic factor) in the brain, which stimulates the production of neuronal stem cells and repairs neuron connections that have been damaged, potentially contributing to much-dreaded brain fog."[22] Your nervous system prefers fat as well, because it's needed by the neurotransmitters in order for them to transmit signals.

The conclusion? To keep your brain healthy and to stay happy you should decrease grain-based carbohydrates and increase healthy fats.

New research also shows that high-carb foods increase the risk for heart problems. During the consumption of foods high in sugar, there appears to be a temporary and sudden dysfunction in the endothelial walls of the arteries.

Dr. Michael Schechter, a senior cardiologist and associate professor of cardiology at the Sackler Faculty of Medicine, Tel Aviv University, found enormous peaks in arterial stress in high-glycemic-index groups. "We knew high glycemic foods were bad for the heart," he says. "Now we have a mechanism that shows how. Foods like cornflakes, white bread, fries, and sweetened soda all put undue stress on our arteries. We've explained for the first time how high-glycemic carbs can affect the progression of heart disease."[23]

Protein

Protein is the fundamental building block for life and plays a key role in the Functional Ketogenic Gut Repair Program.

Protein is required to build new tissue, replicate DNA, catalyze metabolic functions, transport molecules, and help create hormones, antibodies, enzymes, and other compounds. Proteins are made up of chains of amino acids, nine of which are essential. Which mean you must get them from external sources since the body can't make them. A "complete" protein, such as beef, has all of these essential amino acids. However, your body doesn't need a 16-ounce or 500 g steak. Yes, we must have protein, but only in small amounts at one time—2–4 ounces or 60–120 g per serving is a healthy average, based on a person's body size, age, and physical state. A large man may need a little more.

Unfortunately, not all protein is created equal. Vegetarian/vegan sources of protein, whether rice and beans or soy, come with serious health implications because they inhibit digestion and impair absorption. Long term, they lead to deficiencies in the human body that can take a significant toll on overall well-being.

But I've Heard That Meat Isn't Good for Me . . .

You may have heard about the book *The China Study: Startling Implications for Diet, Weight Loss, and Long-Term Health*, written by T. Colin Campbell, PhD, professor emeritus of the division of Nutritional Sciences of Cornell University, published in 2005. *The China Study*, which examines the link between chronic illnesses such as cardiovascular disease and cancer and the consumption of animal-based versus vegetable-based diets, concluded that people who ate diets high in animal foods were likely to have more chronic diseases and higher mortality rates than people who ate plant-based diets.

Many people have taken this book's findings as facts—but are they?

Results of *The China Study* have been strongly contested, largely based on the inclusion of faulty data that does not support the study's hypothesis and the exclusion of data that contradicts it. For example, Campbell and the other authors neglect to identify protein types and dozens of environmental, constitutional, and other dietary and lifestyle factors. Also, the very design of the study on which *The China Study* is based appears to be flawed. The study included questionnaires, food intake as measured by dietary composition tables (rather than what was actually consumed), and used comparative mortality data from the areas in China studied that were drawn from records dated a decade earlier than the 1983 study itself. This is not appropriate data collection.

In *The Protein Debate,* a dialogue about *The China Study* between the study's author, T. Colin Campbell, and Loren Cordain, PhD, a professor in the division of Health and Human Sciences at Colorado State University, Professor Cordain posits that a diet low in animal protein is inconsistent with our evolutionary history.[24] He supports his view with scientific evidence showing that the intake of lean animal protein may in fact *reduce* the risk of the chronic conditions mentioned in *The China Study.*

Cordain, author of *The Paleo Diet*, also points out that our genes have been engineered by a process of natural selection over thousands of years. For example: our ancient ancestors consumed adequate amounts of vitamin C in their diets. As a result, a series of mutations inactivated the functional gene that allows an enzyme (L-Gulono-γ-lactone oxidase) to convert glucose to vitamin C. Consequently, humans now require vitamin C supplementation.

Basically, Campbell's claim that dietary protein should only be 10 percent per day of energy intake for both sexes at all ages seems based in mere speculation and not science. Fundamental physiological nutrient needs vary, depending upon the stage of development, gender, age, and level of fitness. The average American diet already consists of 11–22 percent dietary protein per day. Most of this protein is meat-based, and the meat itself is feedlot-raised, grain-fed, hormone and antibiotic-laden, and unsustainably raised, containing a higher bad fat content that has already been linked to disease. Compare that to the 19–35 percent recommended protein levels on the Paleo diet (consisting of vastly different kinds of protein, usually local, organic, grass-fed, and/or wild). Taking a scientific perspective, for Campbell's 10 percent protein claim to be true, our human ancestors would need to have consumed a low-protein diet over many thousands of years for the human body to have made the required genetic adaptations to exist on so little protein. Ethnographic and fossil evidence of man's evolutionary eating habits and energy needs clearly contradict this.

Another argument in the "low-protein is better" debate is the fact that several studies show that high-protein diets appear to bear a relationship to several types of cancer—in particular, colorectal cancer. And yet vegetarians and vegans are no better off than their meat-eating brethren in this regard. A large cohort study of nearly 11,000 men and women in the United Kingdom did not show a significant difference in colorectal cancer risk between vegetarians/vegans and people who ate meat.[25]

Finally, Cordain's strongest argument in support of the benefits of animal protein from an evolutionary perspective is compelling. Without the consumption of the protein, fat, minerals, and vitamins in meat, the human brain would have been unable to meet the energy needs required to evolve and grow over a few million years into what it is today.

A CASE STUDY

"Alice" was 29 years old. Her chief complaints were fatigue, weight gain, and bloated stomach, with bouts of gas that were uncomfortable. She also bruised easily. I did a full Traditional Chinese Medical history, asking questions about her nutrition and lifestyle. She'd been a vegetarian for eight years. She did eat cheese, craved sweets, and ate processed foods several times a week. She complained of afternoon energy crashes and reached for sweets and caffeine to make it through the day. She ate salads four times a week and loved to eat breads and pastas that helped her feel full.

Barely able to work, unable to exercise, too tired to socialize, she was feeling desperate.

I never pressure anyone into eating anything to which they are averse, but meat happened to be one of the foods that would help strengthen and build her blood. After I shared my personal vegetarian story with her, she became open to drinking bone broth. She agreed to stop gluten and dairy and eat only lightly cooked, stir-fried, and steamed vegetables and avoid salads for two months. She agreed to switch from coffee to green tea, cut back on sweets, take a short walk in nature at least twice each week, and go to bed earlier.

Within five days, her bloating and gas were gone. In two weeks, she'd lost three pounds and reported feeling lighter. In four weeks, she began to exercise and felt like she was coming back to life. On her own, she decided to eat two bites of beef, reporting that her body really liked it. She began to branch out by eating a tiny bit of fish and buffalo. I suggested enzymes to help with the digestion of the meat she was introducing, and she complied. In two months, her energy was about 80 percent back, she'd lost almost 10 pounds, and she felt like she was on the right track.

Alice's story is the perfect example of food as medicine. She's still mostly a vegetarian but adds bone broth to her nutritional plan a few days a month and eats some meat one to three times a week. She is almost completely off sugar and no longer has energy crashes in the afternoon. As an added bonus, she was happy to report the return of her libido energy.

Bottom line, meat protein is not the problem. The problem is the fact that most Westerners have developed an unnatural dependency on carbohydrates. We've spent our entire lives forcing our bodies to adapt to something they were never designed to adapt to. And the reason why your doctors never told you this is because most Western doctors have little to no training in nutrition. And whatever training nutritionists have is likely funded and developed by the industrial processed-food complex.

Today, food is as much about money as sustenance. Gigantic planta-tions of monocrop grains dependent on fossil-fuel-based fertilizers are processed and packaged or force-fed to animals in extreme confinement in vast filthy feedlots. The economic fact is that grain carbohydrates and corn-fed animals, such as beef, pork, and lamb, and grain-fed poultry, such as chicken and turkey, supply the cheapest nutrients for the highest profit.[26] Grains provide a basic nutritional foundation and play a primary role in supporting most of the world's population. They're relatively inexpensive per calorie, can be grown and harvested in huge volumes, and can be stored for long periods of time. They just make good cents.

The food industry has also been developing "new food" for quite some time. Since 1990, more than 100,000 processed foods have been introduced to the market. At least a quarter of them are "nutritionally enhanced" in order to claim health-promoting properties such as "low fat," "cholesterol free," or "higher in calcium."[27] This frightening fact supports this book's urgent move to empower and educate you to change what, how, and when you eat.

Let vegetables fill your carbohydrate needs, let fats provide energy/fuel, and use proteins as building blocks for strong, healthy tissues. Once you shift to an optimized functional ketogenic gut repair nutritional plan, it can take anywhere from three days to up to two months to convert your metabolism from carbohydrate junkie to fat-burning powerhouse. I consider a functional ketogenic gut repair plan a therapeutic diet that can be extremely beneficial and safe for long periods of time—a diet that is especially wonderful during gut repair.

You may feel tired for a few days as you wean your body from its carbo-hydrate addiction. You may experience flu-like symptoms. See chapter 14, "Supplements: Discover and Discern What Is Best" for more details. You may have sugar cravings during the transition period. But you likely have those already. (Consider using the herb Gymnema sylvestre, commonly used to curb carbohydrate cravings and help regulate healthy blood sugar levels.) And when you crave sweets, reach for a healthy fat such as avocado, coconut butter, raw coconut chunks, or turn to a scrumptious recipe in this book. (See Chapter 10, "Sugar Cravings and How to Stop Them Fast" for more practical tips on curbing those cravings.)

There is light at the end of the tunnel in the form of vibrant health!

Chapter 7

Gluten, Phytates, and Lectins. Oh My!

Grains are often touted as the basis of a healthy diet. Yet, as we've seen, this is far from the truth. There are three main reasons for this: the overabundance of carbohydrates in all grains; the presence of anti-nutrient phytates and lectins that negate grains' potential nutritional benefit; and the insidious damage that the gluten in some grains causes for many people.

The media and food industry have led us to believe that grains, nuts, seeds, legumes, and beans are full of nutrients that are good for the body and therefore should be eaten often. But this is not the full truth. All grains, nuts, seeds, legumes, and beans store phosphorus as phytic acid. When phytic acid is bound to a mineral in the seed, it's known as phytate. Grains, seeds, nuts, legumes, and beans contain phytates, which are considered anti-nutrients because they bind to minerals and render them mostly bio-unavailable.

In other words, the absorption of essential minerals such as calcium, iron, magnesium, and zinc is blocked in the presence of phytates. Grains, legumes, and other seeds are also the best known sources of naturally occurring enzyme inhibitors. These anti-enzyme compounds, such as potent trypsin inhibitors and alpha amylase inhibitors, are one of the reasons most people need to supplement with digestive enzymes nowadays. So, it's best to avoid these foods.

Grains, nuts, seeds, legumes, and beans also contain pro-inflammatory lectins that resist digestive enzymes and stomach acid. Mother Nature made them this way for a reason—lectins provide a defense against microorganisms and insects. They're sugar-binding proteins that weaken digestion by adhering to the cells in the lining of the small intestine. Their stickiness is similar to gluten in the way they clog the digestive tract and block absorption. Humans just can't digest lectins.

So what happens to these undigested proteins? They enter the blood and cause the immune system to react. Why does that happen?

Well, foods we don't digest, we make antibodies to fight. And almost everyone has antibodies to some kind of food lectin. Lectins can damage the intestinal lining little by little. Reactions can vary and even be unnoticeable for many years. But lectin damage can occur over time and become a disease process. Normally, the body would repair this. But lectins also hinder the natural cell repair of the intestinal lining, leading to leaky gut over time.

But What about Rice?

How do we reconcile the elimination of rice from the ketogenic way of eating when rice is a dietary staple in China and other parts of the Far East?

The first documented evidence of rice as a crop was a decree by the Chinese emperor back in 2800 B.C. approving it as suitable for sustaining the existence of a growing, no-longer-nomadic society. It wasn't on anyone's health benefit list or even compatible with their genetics and digestive systems. But it would serve as an inexpensive food solution.

That said, the rice grown so long ago was very different from the grain we know today. Historically, the sowing, harvesting, and milling of rice were done by hand—a very laborious process. Modern industrial processing now polishes rice, removing the bran to make white rice that is reduced in protein content and devoid of vitamins and minerals, such as vitamin B and thiamine (although in the presence of phytic acid and lectins, many of the nutrients are not absorbable anyway).

But a low nutrient level is not the only difference between rice, then and now. Modern cultivation methods cause exposure to water-borne pollutants from bedrock and industrial waste, including elevated levels of arsenic and cadmium due to pesticides, fertilizer, and preservatives.[28] These toxins in the water are drawn into the rice plants through their roots. The outer hull of rice—the brown bran—accumulates arsenic, causing brown rice to contain even higher levels of arsenic than white rice with the hull removed—perhaps 10 times as high, according to the U.S. Department of Agriculture.

Some of the highest concentrations of arsenic in rice have been found in the Mississippi River floodplain in the southern United States, where three-quarters of US rice is grown. Even at low levels, arsenic can adversely affect health. It can be detected in the urine of people who frequently consume rice, and is known to cause skin, bladder, and lung cancer. The FDA is currently evaluating whether to set a safe level for the amount of arsenic in food. Think about that the next time you're tempted to include rice in your diet.

But what about other unrefined grains, you ask? Aren't they better for us? Well … um … no. They're advertised as being better for us, but they also contain anti-nutrients and lectins. **Please note:** Not all lectins are bad for you. There are some healthy ones that help with basic cell function and can decrease the incidence of certain diseases. But the lectins found in grains and legumes are not good for humans at all. We're simply not equipped to digest them.

So, what can you do?

If you choose to continue eating these foods, there are a few tricks you should understand. Soaking, sprouting, fermenting, and cooking can help to decrease the lectin content. Vegans, vegetarians, and raw foodists tout the benefits of sprouted grains, nuts, and seeds for good reason. And once the gut-repair phase of your nutritional plan is complete, seeds and nuts can supply good fats and nutrients—but only if they're first soaked in water and sprouted, a process that tricks them into releasing their enzymatic coating of phytates in prep-aration for germination, consequently making them more bioavailable to our human digestive systems.

The Particular Perils of Gluten Grains

Most people have come to believe that whole grains are a "health food." However, I've had the opportunity to personally witness their ill effects. The primary culprit in this "health food" fraud is gluten-containing grains, including wheat, barley, rye, spelt, and khorasan wheat. (Khorasan wheat is also known as Egyptian wheat, Polish wheat, camel's wheat, or Kamut®). The gluten in these grains contains a protein known as gliadin, which is the trigger for celiac disease. There are likely more proteins in gluten that cause problems, but we don't have reliable testing for them yet. Oats do not usually contain gliadin. But they are often harvested and processed by the same equipment used for processing gliadin-containing grains. Oats also contain proteins that are similar to gliadins and therefore poten-tially cross-reactive. This means the oat protein is similar enough to the gliadin protein that your body may respond as if it were gluten.

As a result of consuming these "health foods," a growing number of people are suffering from celiac disease (CD) or non-celiac gluten sensi-tivity (NCGS). Celiac disease attacks the intestines as well as other vital organs and tissues, while non-celiac gluten sensitivity causes inflam-mation and damage to other parts of the body. Approximately one in

133 Americans suffer from diagnosed celiac disease. However, a growing number of people with celiac disease and NCGS go undiagnosed each year. One reason is that symptoms can be vague and transient, and most doctors are unaware of new tests that are now available. Although this testing is not perfect, thanks to researchers like Dr. Aristo Vojdaniand at Cyrex Labs we've made huge leaps forward.

Still Don't Believe That Gluten Is All That Bad?

Many people rightfully question how a food that's been consumed for thousands of years can be harming our bodies now. The answer is complex. First, we must understand exactly what gluten is and from where it comes. The gliadin protein in gluten has a strong binding quality. If you've ever baked bread, you know about the elastic consistency of dough. It has a high level of sticky, gooey adhesiveness. Yes, the bread tastes wonderful. But imagine that stickiness in your intestines. Not so great.

While gluten grains are not acutely poisonous (unless you have celiac disease), they can be chronically degenerative. There is a strong correlation between the introduction of grains into the human diet and the emergence of chronic degenerative diseases such as obesity, cardiovascular disease, osteoporosis, diabetes, cancer, and thyroid/endocrine disorders, to name a few.[29]

The Fertile Crescent (comprising present-day Egypt, Iraq, Kuwait, Syria, Israel/Palestine, northeast Africa, the Ethiopian highlands, Turkey, and Iran) was one of the first regions to domesticate and cultivate wheat. And research on mummified bodies proves that they had degenerative diseases such as osteoporosis and heart disease.

In what's known as the "Egyptian Mummy Diet Paradox," entombed Egyptians dating back as far as 3,500 years were found to have heart disease and atherosclerosis (hardening of the arteries). An April 2011 report in the *Journal of the American College of Cardiology on cardiovascular imaging* showed via CT scanning that nearly half of ancient Egyptian mummies with identifiable cardiovascular structures had evidence of atherosclerosis.[30] The heart, aorta, and blood vessels of the legs all showed calcification. Modern Americans and Europeans examined by CT (computerized tomography) show similar calcification due to atherosclerosis. Dr. Daniel Auer, an integrative health practitioner and "medical detective" in the US, has set forward the hypothesis that carbohydrate intake was the cause.

And it's not just ancient Egyptians and modern Westerners that carbs have affected. Both Greek and Roman Empires were built on the backs of Egyptian wheat. Around A.D. 250, the Greek physician Aretaeus of

Cappadocia wrote detailed descriptions of an unnamed disease. When describing his patients, he referred to them as *koiliakos*, which meant "suffering in the bowels." He recommended to his patients suffering from this condition that they change their diet, but he didn't connect it to grains. This is possibly one of the earliest accounts of what would later be known as celiac disease; therefore, it's not a new disease stemming from GMO wheat as many hypothesize.

In 1843, a physician named Stanislas Tanchou, speaking at the Paris Medical Society Conference, claimed he could predict cancer rates in major European cities over the next 50 years based on the percentage of grains being consumed in each major city. And over time, his predictions have proven to be correct. Cancer rates are indeed highest in the cities with the highest grain consumption. In contrast to this, in populations where grains are not consumed, cancer does not exist.[31]

Gluten is "gooey" food that's not good for anyone. The unfortunate truth is that it not only impairs your health, it targets your brain. "Gluten sensitivity should be considered as a state of heightened immunologic responsiveness to ingested gluten proteins in genetically predisposed individuals. The brain seems to be particularly vulnerable."[32] It is now evident that gluten damages the brain and nervous tissue more than any other tissue in the body.[33] For a more in-depth study of the vital role that nutrition and the brain have on your overall health, please read Dr. Datis Kharrazian's book *Why Isn't My Brain Working?*

NCGS (non-celiac gluten sensitivity) has been shown to be a trigger in cerebellar disease,[34] cognitive impairment,[35] multiple sclerosis,[36] ataxia or impaired muscle coordination,[37] general neurological impairment,[38] sensory ganglionopathy,[39] psychiatric disorders,[40] migraines,[41] and restless leg syndrome.[42] The protein structures of gluten are similar to nervous system tissues. When you have sensitivity to gluten, your immune system produces gluten antibodies that tag these proteins for destruction. Because of the similarity of gluten proteins to your nervous system tissues, your body may make antibodies to your nervous tissues, thus becoming an autoimmune reaction against your brain and nervous system tissues.[43] This is known as tissue mimicry.

Known as a "silent killer," gluten is sneaky! Day after day, week after week, year after year, it negatively impacts the immune, neurological, muscular/skeletal, cardiovascular, and endocrine systems. And you may not know it until you're diagnosed with a stroke, a heart attack due to hypoperfusion (reduced blood flow), depression, diabetes, gallstones, a ruptured appendix, cancer, Hashimoto's thyroiditis, uterine fibroids, migraines, arthritis, multiple sclerosis, or lupus, to name the more prominent conditions. As an article in *The New England Journal of Medicine* states: "Celiac disease is one of the most common lifelong disorders in both Europe and the United States. The clinical presentation of this condition can range from the typical syndrome of malabsorption (chronic diarrhea, weight loss, and abdominal distention) to symptoms and conditions that can affect any organ system."[44]

Take note: *any organ system!* Celiac disease is considered to be an autoimmune disorder. "Celiac disease 'out of the intestine' is even more frequent than celiac disease 'within the intestine.'"[45] *This means that gluten-sensitivity disease patterns can appear as an autoimmune response affecting any organ system.*

In 2001, the British medical journal *The Lancet* published a study titled, "Mortality in Patients with Celiac Disease and their Relatives: A Cohort Study." The study comprised 1,072 adult celiacs and 3,384 first-degree relatives. The standardized mortality ratio was 2.0 (200 percent) with a 20-plus-year follow-up, meaning that people with celiac disease were two times more likely to die before their same-age peers.[46] Many of their family members carried the gene for celiac disease, or NCGS.

And diet and lifestyle can turn those genes on or off—an effect studied in the fascinating field called *epigenetics*. If people carrying the gene eat foods that trigger autoimmune challenges (gluten, milk, eggs, sugar, soy, corn, oats, or any grain cross-reactive foods), make poor lifestyle choices, and have high-stress lifestyles, they too will suffer.

Epigenetics is the study of changes in gene activity caused by environmental and nutritional factors rather than by changes in the DNA sequence. The impact of epigenetics on health is well described in *The Biology of Belief* by Dr. Bruce Lipton and *Pottenger's Prophecy: How Food Resets Genes for Wellness or Illness* by Gray Graham, Deborah Kesten, and Larry Scherwitz. Environmental chemicals, nutrition, stress, and even emotions and thought patterns all have the power to alter the expression of genes, thus creating a foundation for wellness or for disease. What you eat, how you live, and what you think strongly influence your own life and the lives of your descendants for many generations. According to *Pottenger's Prophecy*, it can take approximately three generations to alter an unhealthy genetic expression. Now is the best time to begin!

A Loving Note to Parents

You may think you and your children are just fine and have no food sensitivities, but if you are what you eat, then in 10 years your health will directly reflect your nutritional choices now. And if you or your children already have poor balance or coordination, headaches, mood disorders (depression, anxiety), learning, memory, or attention disabilities (ADD, ADHD), asthma, skin problems (rashes, eczema, psoriasis, acne), digestive troubles (gas, bloating, diarrhea, constipation, failure to thrive), cardiovascular challenges (high blood pressure, high cholesterol, high homocysteine, high CRP), thyroid imbalance (fatigue, hair loss, dry skin, weight fluctuations, brain fog, thinning outer edges of eyebrows), immune impairment (chronic or recurrent infections like bronchitis, sinusitis, slow healing, ear or throat infections, or seasonal allergies), you're in trouble NOW.

Getting your child on a gluten-free diet may well prevent their future suffering and early death. Autoimmune diseases are 10 times more common in those with celiac disease than in the general population.[47] And that's not all. The duration of exposure to gluten increases the risk of developing an autoimmune disease for those who have celiac disease or NCGS (non-celiac gluten sensitivity). The journal *Gastroenterology*[48] states that only 1 in 20 celiac patients who stop gluten exposure at age two go on to develop an autoimmune disorder. But for those children who continue gluten exposure until age 20, the risk jumps to *1 in 3*! Non-adherence to a gluten-free diet ("non-adherence" is defined as eating gluten once per month) increases the relative risk of death by 600 percent.[49]

Now do I have your attention?

If you can only make one change to your diet and your children's diets, stop eating all gluten and glutenous grains, including wheat, barley, rye, spelt, and khorasan wheat. By eliminating gluten and increasing your vegetable consumption, you'll be increasing the quality and length of your life and the lives of your children.

Chapter 8

Dangers of Dairy and the Sad Story of Soy

You may be surprised that I use the words "danger" and "dairy" in the same sentence. After all, in America, you've likely seen dozens of celebrities sporting milk moustaches asking, "Got Milk?" and thousands of ads on TV declaring that milk is a health drink that "builds strong bodies." We've been told it's great for bones and teeth and that we should have at least three servings per day. There's nothing so healthy as milk. It's what we give our kids. It's what Americans drink along with their apple pie. Right?

My own mother argued for the wholesomeness of milk, asking me, "Why would the Dairy Council promote something that isn't good for us?" I sat her down and gave her several answers, which I'll share with you here.

First, it's very difficult to prove something is bad for us, especially in the face of entrenched cultural and economic interests. Consider how long it took to educate and convince the public about the dangers of tobacco smoking. And millions of people still smoke! Someone who wishes to believe dairy is good for them will find abundant confirmation and reinforcement for their belief in the popular media and fast-food culture. Even the FDA assures us that dairy foods are safe. As a result, people who are allergic to dairy may not even recognize that there's an association between dairy and their symptoms.

Moreover, there are huge economic interests in dairy farming and production. America's dairy industry is more than milk; it's jobs and economic activity. There are about 51,000 dairy farms in the United States. "Without dairy farmers, local tax bases would look very different and that would affect schools, local businesses, and the food supply—it would also affect the natural landscape and wide-open spaces that farmers help provide."[50]

I'm happy to stimulate and support the economy, but not by risking the health and well-being of our population. Cow's milk is excellent for baby cows, but not for humans. Consider this: Humans are the *only* animal species in existence that drinks another species' milk. Granted, cow's milk is not acutely poisonous, and it can support life. But there are long-term degenerative health consequences, because there's a vast physiological difference between cows and humans. Cows have four stomach chambers, and smaller breeds grow to be 600–1,000 pounds. Larger breeds reach 1,400–2,400 pounds. Humans have only one stomach, and we hope to never get even close to 600 pounds.

Between the ages of two and five, children lose the ability to produce the enzymes necessary to digest milk protein, whether pasteurized or raw.[51] As we've seen before, whatever we don't properly digest can cause immune challenges. The Wexner Medical Center of Ohio State University reports that *30 to 50 million Americans (adults and children) are lactose intolerant.* Lactose intolerance is caused by the absence of the enzyme lactase, which is necessary to digest the milk sugar called lactose. When sour milk curdles, it separates into a solid and a liquid portion. The solid part is casein, the dominant protein in milk; the liquid part is called whey, which is mostly water and lactose. People can have intolerance or true allergies to one or both.

According to the National Digestive Diseases Information Clearinghouse (NDDIC), a service of the National Institute of Diabetes and Digestive and Kidney Diseases (NIDDK), National Institutes of Health (NIH), "primary lactase deficiency develops over time and begins after about age two, when the body begins to produce less lactase. Most children who have lactase deficiency do not experience symptoms of lactose intolerance until late adolescence or adulthood."[52]

Lactose intolerance is different from a true milk allergy but is related to it and can lead to a true milk allergy over time. In a true milk allergy, the immune system is already reacting to casein (milk protein). The NIDDK goes on to state that "secondary lactase deficiency results from injury to the small intestine that occurs with severe diarrheal illness, celiac disease, Crohn's disease, or chemotherapy."[53]

To that list I would add non-celiac gluten sensitivity, exposure to toxins and heavy metals that pass through the placenta to the fetus, inadequate breastfeeding in infancy, plus other food allergens and sensitivities that lead to damaged villi in the small intestine, all of which compromise GI health and immune function.

Lactose is present in varying amounts in the milk of all species that produce it (cow, goat, sheep, and human) and to some degree in all milk products—butter, cream, buttermilk, cheese, cottage cheese, yogurt, and ice cream. Whey is very high in lactose and is thus a high-allergen food, especially for people with celiac disease and NCGS. A study published in the journal *Food and Nutrition Sciences* reveals that casein caused the next highest cross-reactivity immune response in individuals with celiac disease, compared with other non-gliadin food antigens. This was followed by yeast, casomorphins (which are peptides, or protein fragments, derived from the digestion of milk protein), oat cultivar, and fresh corn.[54]

THE SCIENCE
BOVINE LEUKEMIA VIRUS (BLV)

Cattle carry hundreds of viruses and bacteria foreign to humans. When we ingest their milk—pasteurized or raw—we're allowing our immune systems to be assaulted with these bovine viruses and bacteria. Bovine leukemia virus (BLV) is a retrovirus that is closely related to the human T-lymphotropic virus type 1 (HTLV-1). The USDA found a high prevalence of the virus in US cattle, but this problem is also well known in Europe.

As part of a 2007 dairy study in the US, bulk tank milk was collected from 534 operations with 30 or more dairy cows and tested with an enzyme-linked immunosorbent assay for the presence of antibodies against BLV. Results showed that 83.9 percent of US dairy operations were positive for BLV.[55] Under natural conditions, the disease is transmitted mainly by milk to the calf, and there is no treatment available. Studies to detect human pathogenicity in farm workers who drank the raw milk were negative, which shows only that humans don't contract BLV. One recent study has found a connection between BLV and breast cancer. To illustrate the potential for cross-species disease vectors, studies have shown that butchers and slaughterhouse workers are more vulnerable to certain cancers.

One prevalent myth is that cow's milk is a good source of calcium. Debunking the calcium myth is quite simple. Basic chemistry shows us that cow's milk contains phosphorus, which binds to calcium, rendering it unavailable for absorption. Some calcium is absorbable from cow's milk, but most is not. Large mammals, such as cows and elephants, get their calcium from grasses and other plants. But most commercial dairy cows aren't pasture-raised anymore; now they're fed grain and a variety of junk—including (I kid you not) candy—supplemented with hormones, synthetic vitamins, and minerals. We've already noted that gluten from grain has a negative effect on absorption rates and bone density. Nearly a third of all North American women will develop osteoporosis that results in a bone fracture.

Not surprisingly, cows exclusively fed grain are also now breaking their bones at an alarming rate.

Drinking milk actually *increases* the risk of fracture in humans. Diane Feskanich, ScD. Assistant Professor at Harvard Medical School, conducted a 12-year study with 77,761 women aged 34 to 59 years who had never taken calcium supplements. Every two years between 1980 and 1986, they filled out a food-frequency questionnaire and reported their incidence of bone fractures. The findings were stunning: Women who drank two or more glasses of milk per day had a higher risk of hip and forearm fractures than women who consumed one glass or less per week; women who drank at least two glasses of milk per day showed a 45 percent increase in hip fractures compared with those who rarely drank milk.[56] This suggests that instead of milk consumption protecting women against osteoporotic fractures it actually increases the likelihood of that happening.

A 1993 Finnish study also found that childhood consumption of bovine dairy products increased the risk of insulin-dependent diabetes mellitus.[57] Beta-lactoglobulin, a protein in cow's milk, is similar to glycodelin found in humans. Glycodelin impacts immune function as a T-cell modulator. An infant's intestines are not fully "closed"—their tight junctions are not yet sealed—essentially meaning that they are born with a leaky gut. Therefore, proteins leak through the gaps in the small intestine, intro-ducing foreign bovine milk proteins—food antigens—into the blood. The immune system becomes alarmed and confused. Anti-beta-lactoglobulin cross-reacts to glycodelin, causing babies to make antibodies that also attack glycodelin, an essential protein that helps train the immune system. The T-cell regulation of beta cells is negatively impacted. The mistuned immune system then mistakenly destroys insulin-producing pancreatic cells, leading to Type 1 diabetes.[58]

There is also controversy in the medical literature about xanthine oxidase, a potential source of free radicals found in milk, which at high levels is linked to endothelial dysfunction and cardiovascular disease.[59]

In addition, many investigators have found a link between multiple sclerosis and milk consumption.[60]

Besides the long list of associated diseases, milk is also responsible for gastrointestinal, respiratory,[61] behavioral, and skin disorders. Dr. Sami Bahna, chief of allergy and immunology at Louisiana State University Health Sciences Center in Shreveport, states that: "Pediatricians often recognize the link between gastrointestinal or skin manifestations of this allergy, but many are unaware of the link to asthma symptoms. In fact, although it's not frequent, asthma can be the only manifestation of a cow's milk allergy in some children."[62]

Dr. William Sears, a well-known pediatrician and author, says "milk allergies cause repeated colds and ear infections."[63, 64] So despite what the dairy marketing associations want you to believe, the evidence shows that milk doesn't actually "do a body good." To add insult to injury, the dairy industry petitioned the FDA to approve aspartame (an artificial, non-saccharide sweetener used as a sugar substitute) as a hidden, unlabeled additive in milk, yogurt, eggnog, and cream![65]

Yet another reason to be wary of dairy.

The (Sadly) Successful Soy Story

In the last 50 years, the commercial rise of soy as a human food and animal feed source has been nothing less than phenomenal. By the year 1997, the US retail soy-foods industry was bringing in revenues around $1 billion per annum. In 2013, the total was $4.5 billion, continuing an 11-year trend of 15 percent average annual increases. According to the United Soybean Board's 2004–2005 report, *Consumer Attitudes About Nutrition*, 25 percent of Americans consume soy foods or beverages at least once per week, and 74 percent view soy products as healthy.[66]

Fractionated soy, including soy flour, textured soy protein, partially hydrogenated soybean oil, and soy protein isolate—none of which can be found in the traditional Japanese diet—are found in commercial soy cheese, milk, margarine, vegetable oils, burgers and hot dogs, baby formula, and flour, to name just a few products now on the market. Alongside corn, soy derivatives have also become a major ingredient in fast foods and prepackaged frozen meals.

Dramatic growth in soy product popularity followed the FDA approval of a health claim linking soy with heart disease reduction.[67] And yet, according to Julia R. Barrett, M.D., M.P.H., a senior clinical consultant for Biologics Consulting in Denver, "Soybeans are a major allergen, and a significant percentage of children who are sensitive to dairy are also sensitive to soy."

In her article "The Science of Soy: What Do We Really Know?" Barrett continues: "Isoflavones belong to a class of compounds generally known as phytoestrogens, plant compounds that have estrogen-like structures. Soy isoflavones have been linked with numerous health effects, but the strength of the relationships and whether the effects are beneficial are strongly debated."[68]

Barrett asserts that these weak estrogens can act as agonists, partial agonists, or antagonists to endogenous estrogens (like estradiol) and xenoestrogens (fake estrogens from plastics) at estrogen receptors. The dominant isoflavone in soy is genistein; the others are daidzein and glycitein. Referencing Retha R. Newbold, a supervisory research biologist at the NIEHS, she writes: "Concerns about genistein's effects on reproduction and development are due in part to her extensive research in mice. Newbold believes caution is warranted, because her studies—and others—have shown that genistein has such effects as inducing uterine adenocarcinoma (cancer that originates in gland or organ tissue) in mice and premature puberty in rats."

In addition, a study led by biologist Wendy Jefferson in Newbold's laboratory, published in the October 2005 issue of *Biology of Reproduction,* linked genistein with effects such as abnormal estrous cycle, altered ovarian function, and infertility in mice.

Modern processed soy foods often have high levels of MSG, fluoride, and aluminum, which are toxic to the nervous system. *Infant formulas based on soy protein isolate contain 100 times more aluminum than is found in breast milk.*[69] At least two categories of carcinogens are formed during the processing of both organic and conventional soy—lysinealanines and nitrosamines. Infant soy formulas contain high levels of isoflavones, which are known to cause endocrine disruption.[70] On average, infants fed soy formula have been shown to ingest up to 11 times the amount of genistein proven to cause hormonal effects in adults.[71] New Zealand toxicologist Mike Fitzpatrick estimates that an infant fed exclusively soy formula receives the estrogenic equivalent of at least five birth control pills per day.

Fitzpatrick also found that a serving of soy food provides up to three times the goitrogenic (thyroid-inhibiting) potency of the pharmaceutical thyroid-inhibiting drugs methimazole and 6-propylthiouracil.[72] Every single cell in your body requires thyroid hormone in order to function properly, and the thyroid-hormone receptor is located in the DNA of each of your cells. In order to heal your gut, you must have proper thyroid function, and your cells must have thyroid hormones.

So, you ask, what about all those millions of healthy Asians who consume soy products on a daily basis? Well, the natural and fermented soy components of the traditional Japanese diet bear no resemblance to the unfermented soy derivatives found in the American diet. Even fermented soy (such as tempeh or miso) is barely fermented in the United States— typically for just a few days or weeks, whereas in Asia, soy is fermented for months or years. (The beneficial aspect of fermented soy products comes from consuming the bacteria responsible for fermentation, rather than the soy itself.) Not only is unfermented soy nearly indigestible, it is also estrogenic (increases estrogen) and goitrogenic (stops thyroid function) and reduces testosterone in both men and women.[73]

Chapter 9

Sugar—Not So Sweet?

Most of us have been raised on a carbohydrate-based diet, which means we're slaves to glucose. As your body digests starches, glucose is the result. You're probably familiar with the terms blood glucose or blood sugar? That's simply the measure of glucose in your bloodstream as your body transports it. And insulin is the hormone that helps to move glucose from your blood into your cells for energy and storage.

We may be slaves to other forms of sugar, too, including fructose, found in fruit. After decades of eating grains and sugars, being exposed to chemicals, pesticides, synthetic food additives, and worn down by emotional stress, most of us are likely experiencing some degree of adrenal fatigue, more accurately known as "hypothalamic-pituitary-adrenal (HPA) axis syndrome." We're also heavily prone to hypoglycemia, insulin resistance, and diabetes.

If you don't eat every few hours, do you get cranky or hangry (hungry and angry)? Do you experience mood swings, headaches, brain fog, fatigue, sugar cravings, trouble sleeping, or low productivity? Do you reach for stimulants like coffee, tea, sugar, and chocolate just to get through those mid-morning and mid-afternoon slumps? If so, it's really quite simple: You're responding to your body's addiction to sugar. Numerous researchers have hypothesized that excess fructose consumption is a primary cause of insulin resistance and obesity[74]—alongside elevated LDL cholesterol and triglycerides—leading to metabolic syndrome.[75] That's right, it's the sugar—not the good fats—that increase your cholesterol.

Americans, Europeans, Central and South Americans, and Asians eat a ton of sugar. Sugar has spread all across the world. Refined white cane sugar, raw sugar, fruit sugar, brown sugar, corn sugar, milk sugar, beet sugar, alcohol, monosaccharides, disaccharides, and polysaccharides—the

$100 billion/year sugar industry promotes them all. In the US, we consume an average of 150 pounds per person, per year.[76]

I remember sprinkling white sugar on my Cheerios as a child and dipping strawberries in it. A friend's mom made her sugar sandwiches for lunch. I'm sure you have your own memories of your favorite sweet treats growing up. But for something so yummy tasting, sugar has terrible health consequences and a surprisingly sordid past. To learn more about the dark historical and political past of the economics of sugar (a story that involves wealthy trade empires and opium) please consider reading *Sugar Blues* by William Dufty.

Sugar = Health Havoc

There is mounting evidence that sugar—not fat—is the leading cause of cardiovascular disease, obesity, kidney disease, diabetes, and metabolic syndrome.[77] Sugar can also contribute to other problems, such as migraines, immune system suppression, hyperactivity in children, kidney damage, acidifying the blood, tooth decay, advanced aging, digestive disorders, arthritis, asthma, Candida albicans, decreased blood flow to the heart, food allergies, eczema, atherosclerosis, free radical formation, loss of enzyme function, increased liver and kidney size, brittle tendons, migraines, blood clots, and depression.

Dr. Weston Price, the dentist known for his landmark work *Nutrition and Physical Degeneration,* traveled around the world in the 1930s examining the teeth and skulls of every "primitive" (translate low-tech and isolated) race he could find—First Nations Americans, Swiss Alps villagers, Alaskan Inuits, Australian aboriginal people, Fiji islanders, and more. What he discovered was that when people in previously isolated traditional societies were introduced to Western foods such as white sugar and white flour, within only a few years, they would start experiencing "diseases of civilization"—tooth decay, tuberculosis, arthritis, obesity, and such—at rates comparable to people in more "modern" parts of the world.

Sugar causes insulin resistance, metabolic syndrome, and diabetes. The beta cells in your pancreas produce insulin to help move glucose in your blood into your cells where it can do its job energizing your body. When our cells become resistant to insulin, because of the overabundance of insulin produced to handle the sugar load, it can cause many serious health problems. Basically, your cells no longer accept the insulin and therefore can't move glucose into the cells where it belongs. As your blood glucose levels rise, the pancreas struggles to keep up with the rising demand for more insulin until it is exhausted and can no longer produce enough. Eventually, this can lead to Type 2 diabetes and all of its miserable complications, including painful neuropathy (pain and numbness in peripheral nerves), blindness, kidney failure, heart attack, and slow-healing wounds that lead to gangrene and amputation.

My grandfather lost his foot to diabetes; my son's grandfather lost his leg; and my mother had a slow-healing wound that required weekly care for over 20 months—all of them are sugar and carbohydrate addicts, and all of them are on diabetes medication or now deceased. My dear mother has been recently diagnosed with dementia and Alzheimer's. I spoke with her neurologist, who reported a decrease in the white matter of her brain. We both concluded it was from the long-term high levels of glucose she maintained, even while on her medication.

Speaking of which, taking insulin or metformin does not mean you can safely eat sugar. If you eat a high-sugar and high-carbohydrate diet, you are likely on the path toward insulin resistance, diabetes, or worse.

So please pay attention! Diabetes stinks—and Type 2 diabetes is 100 percent preventable.

No Sugar, No Cancer?

Cancer can be viewed as a "blip" in the DNA of a cell. Scientists know that humans have these little blips all the time. However, when your immune system is healthy and balanced, it immediately recognizes the sick cell and gets rid of it before the "blip" can turn into a full-blown cancerous tumor or disease. Eating sugar, however, throws a monkey wrench into the clean-up process.

Sugar suppresses immune function for four to eight hours, stopping macrophages, a kind of white blood cell, from hunting down and engulfing "blips" and other bad guys. In addition, cancer cells consume six to eight times more sugar than any other cell in your body. So, if you consume sugar, you are feeding the young cancer cells instead of supporting your immune system to eradicate them.

High levels of insulin caused by sugar and carbohydrate consumption are associated with metabolic syndrome. The Standard American Diet (SAD)—high-carbohydrate, high-sugar, and processed foods; low levels of physical activity; and stress-related brain and hormone imbalances—increases the risk of insulin resistance, high blood insulin levels, and therefore cancer.[78] There is also a strong correlation between metabolic syndrome and the chronic inflammation associated with cancers affecting the colon, prostate, pancreas, and (especially) the breasts.

Insulin/insulin-like growth factor (IGF) has been shown to enhance tumor cell growth. And IGF may interfere with cancer therapy, leading to poor treatment outcomes. Not only can cutting sugar out of your diet be a cancer prevention strategy but if you are diagnosed with cancer, it can positively impact your chances of survival.

Other Sugar Issues

Sugar contributes to osteoporosis: In order for calcium to be used by the bones, there must be enough vitamin D3 and magnesium, and a specific ratio of calcium and phosphorus, or the calcium will remain in an unusable form. Sugar depletes our magnesium stores, which can lead to a build-up of unusable calcium in our blood instead of our bones. It further accumulates and is then filtered by our kidneys or gallbladder, where it may become lodged in the form of a stone. Without the usable form of calcium, our bodies register our calcium stores as low and begin to pull calcium from our bones and teeth, possibly leading to osteoporosis.

Sugar causes mineral deficiencies: Sugar ingestion increases mineral deficiencies in the body, especially of chromium, copper, calcium, and magnesium. Chromium is needed as a cofactor for insulin to work. This is why people who have insulin resistance and diabetes from sugar intake may need more chromium.

Sugar has addictive qualities: Sugar releases dopamine in the "reward center" of the brain, which is why you crave it—you're hooked. Plus, like most addicts, moderation doesn't work. Abstinence is your best chance of surviving sugar's powerful allure. Keep reading to learn how to deal with those pesky cravings.

Sugar makes you fat: There is a huge link between childhood obesity and consumption of sugary drinks. One study found that each daily serving of sugar-sweetened beverages was associated with a 60 percent higher risk of obesity.[79]

High-Fructose Corn Syrup

Sucrose used to be the main source of sugar in the US, but then a process was developed that changed the natural fructose in corn into glucose. When synthetic chemicals were added, it changed the glucose into an artificial sweetener—a synthetic kind of high-fructose sweetener known as high-fructose corn syrup (HFCS). In the early 1980s, big corporations like Coke and Pepsi changed their sugar ingredient from cane sugar to HFCS.

Consuming fructose has been shown to raise blood lipids (cholesterol) and cause decreased cell sensitivity to insulin, leading to higher blood sugar levels and obesity.[80] Studies also show that fructose does not satiate humans as effectively as glucose does. In one study, fructose did not lower ghrelin, the hunger hormone, as much as glucose did. Fructose also negatively impacts regional cerebral blood flow (CBF) to several important structures of the brain, including the thalamus (which transmits movement and sensory information) and the hippocampus (which is associated with memory).[81]

The absorption of fructose isn't completely understood. A portion of it is absorbed in a healthy small intestine. But then a portion also travels to the large intestine, where it is fermented by flora. In an unhealthy small intestine, one that is unable to absorb well due to villous atrophy, damage, or leaky gut (in other words, most of us in Western societies like North America), a higher-than-usual portion goes to the large intestine. In the presence of unabsorbed fructose, the colonic flora then produces carbon dioxide, short-chain fatty acids, organic acids, and trace gases.[82] These gases and organic acids in the large intestine cause gastrointestinal symptoms, such as bloating, diarrhea, flatulence, and gastrointestinal pain.[83] If you have the farts, this could be why.

Fruit juices, honey, high-fructose corn syrup, sucrose, and agave syrup are all high in fructose. Unlike glucose, fructose can only be metabolized by your liver. Sugar (especially fructose) metabolism is "dirty," spinning off a chain of messy byproducts that stress the liver, including uric acid, which blocks an enzyme that makes nitric oxide, your body's natural blood pressure regulator. Dr. Robert Lustig, a professor of Pediatrics in the Division of Endocrinology at the University of California, notes that the damaging effect of fructose is similar to that of alcohol.

He discovered that the liver metabolizes fructose similarly to alcohol, promoting insulin resistance, dyslipidemia, and fatty liver. He also discovered that fructose reacts with proteins, forming superoxide free radicals that can result in liver damage. Finally, his studies reveal that fructose "stimulates the hedonic pathway of the brain," leading to addiction.[84] "Fructose induces alterations in both hepatic [liver] metabolisms and central nervous system energy signaling," he writes, "leading to a vicious cycle of excessive consumption and disease consistent with metabolic syndrome."

Bottom line, sugar is a multibillion-dollar industry producing a product that destroys your body's health—and you pay for it in more ways than one.

Chapter 10

Sugar Cravings and
How to Stop Them Fast

Very few people can eat even a healthy sweet treat without noticing more cravings popping up soon afterwards. If you've completed a four-month gut repair program, then it may be okay for you to enjoy some raw healthy desserts in moderation, with the sweet part of these desserts coming from fruit, monk fruit, stevia, cashews, honey, or coconut syrup. But remember, moderation is the key.

If you need an incentive to get off sugar—other than the fact that it's been proven to cause diabetes, obesity, heart disease, and the inflammation that is part of every single disease pattern in the body; feeds cancer like crazy; causes tooth decay; can overload the liver, turning the sugar you just ate into storable fat; and is comprised of "empty calories" with no nutritional value whatsoever — then how about this: Sugar exacerbates other addictions because it activates the same portions of the brain as other drugs (such as cocaine).

Yikes! No wonder you crave sugar.

Sugar is highly addictive, and the brain becomes habituated to it. Sugar and quick-burning carbohydrates that turn to sugar give you a mood lift by releasing the neurotransmitter serotonin. Unfortunately, this quick boost, repeated over time, leads to an overall depletion of serotonin, which directly impacts your mood by making you depressed. No wonder the rate of depression is sky-rocketing in America—we're sugar junkies!

It is actually immaterial which came first—the habit of eating sugar to soothe emotional unease (anxiety, depression, low self-esteem, idea of "reward," filling a void, stuffing feelings), or our brain's neurochemistry, which leads us to seek out stimulation, experiences, nutrition, and satiation, drives that we misinterpret and mistreat by using sugar—the end result is the same: sugar addiction, and the huge number of problems that come with it.

Nutritional Deficiencies

Cravings can come from nutritional deficiencies. Chocolate is one of the most widely reported cravings, and no wonder. About 80 percent of Americans are deficient in a very important macro-mineral that can cause this craving: magnesium. The body needs magnesium for more than 300 biochemical reactions. Other symptoms of magnesium deficiency include anxiety, constipation, high blood pressure, irritability, insomnia, and muscle problems such as cramping.

Sugary foods are the second most commonly reported craving in the West. This one is a little trickier because there are at least five nutrient deficiencies that may cause this craving. They are chromium (which helps to regulate blood sugar levels), carbon (one of the elements from which sugar is made), phosphorus (which helps the body produce energy), sulfur (which helps remove toxins), magnesium (helps with calcium absorption, muscle and brain function), and tryptophan (which helps regulate serotonin).

Cravings for refined carbohydrates—those junky, processed, quick, sugary foods that don't come from nature—can signal a nitrogen deficiency. Nitrogen compounds are an essential component of nucleic acid and protein, and a deficiency may indicate malnutrition due to lack of protein.

If you crave oily and fatty foods, you may be deficient in calcium. Eat some collard greens to boost bioavailable calcium and take vitamin D3.

Finally, if you crave salty foods, you may be low in chloride and/or silicon.

Hormonal Fluctuations

Cravings can come from hormonal fluctuations. Right before menstruation, a woman's estrogen is low, progesterone is on its way down and beta-endorphins are also at their lowest. Beta-endorphin is another neurotransmitter that is released when we eat sugar; the same neurotransmitter is released during exercise and acts as an analgesic and produces the well-known "runner's high" sensation. Exercise can help hormone-driven cravings.

Stress Can Cause Sugar Cravings

Stress causes the release of the hormone cortisol and temporarily dampens hunger, but after the stress has passed, the body ramps up and wants to replenish its nutrient stores. Stress can contribute to poor nutritional habits—some people "stress eat," using food in an attempt to alleviate the discomforts of stress, both physical and emotional. People under stress often crave sugar and carbohydrates.

If the adrenals are tired, then some carbohydrate consumption can be therapeutic. However, if you're reaching for sweets in an attempt to de-stress and find comfort, you're moving in an unhealthy direction.

Food Sensitivities, Leaky Gut, and Cravings

Which came first, the food sensitivity or the leaky gut? Each one leads to the other. There are other causes of leaky gut, but eating foods that you may have a hidden sensitivity to is a common one. Leaky gut occurs when food particles that are only partially digested make their way into the bloodstream through a damaged, inflamed mucosal lining in the digestive tract. The body identifies these food particles as foreign invaders (also known as *antigens*) and launches an immune system attack by sending antibodies after them. The combination of immune complex, antigens, and antibodies in your bloodstream can lead to intense cravings.

Gluten may be at the root of this craving, because it causes both leaky gut and an immune response. Some people misinterpret these cravings as a sweet tooth, when really the sweet cravings are triggered by gluten. If you crave a particular unhealthy food, it is likely you have a sensitivity to it.

Yeast and Candida

Yeast feeds on sugar. You develop an imbalance of yeast when the good bacteria in your intestines and/or vagina are decreased and the bad bacteria and fungi are increased. This is known as *dysbiosis*, and it leads to a yeast overgrowth. This often happens when someone has taken an antibiotic, because antibiotics don't differentiate between bacteria—they just kill them all, including the good ones. Then the bad yeast takes this opportunity to grow.

Yeast loves sugar and will stimulate cravings for it. You can keep the numbers of bad yeast down and good bacteria up by taking professional-grade prebiotics and probiotics, avoiding sugar, and identifying the root cause. You may also have candida if you have even low levels of heavy metal toxicity. This will perpetuate candida growth and sugar cravings.

Note: Candida can actually protect the body from high levels of mercury. If you attempt to kill the yeast without eliminating the root cause—the heavy metal—you will feel sick and never really successfully free yourself from it.

How to Curb Your Sugar Cravings

Here are some ideas to help you when you feel those cravings creeping in:

- Drink a glass of spring water.
- Eat some protein and healthy fat.
- Eat regularly to avoid blood sugar drops, which increase sugar/carb cravings.
- Don't postpone eating. Eat as soon as you feel hungry, or two to three hours after your last meal, depending on your blood sugar and ketogenic status.
- Become a grazer. Eat crunchy veggies, or make raw crunchy veggie chips in a dehydrator.
- Take a dose of digestive bitters. This helps curb sweet cravings quickly, while supporting your digestion.
- Eat some healthy fruit while you wean off the bad sugars. An apple tastes sweet, but it also has fiber and pectin. Try combining it with some nut butters (almond, cashew, coconut, pecan, or hazelnut) to help slow the absorption of its natural sugars. This also helps stabilize your blood sugar.
- Have a cup of peppermint tea. It is slightly sweet and may just do the trick.
- Choose quality over quantity. Rather than gorging on junk food made with highly processed sugars, choose a natural sweet in moderation, such as fresh organic berries or a square of dark chocolate with 75 percent or higher cacao content.
- Exercise. Moving your body will refocus your metabolism and your mind, and exercise releases endorphins. Also, when you get out of the house, you are distancing yourself from the old habits associated with the craving.
- Rid your pantry of junk food. If it's out of sight, it's more likely out of mind.
- Avoid artificial sweeteners. These toxic chemicals are manufactured to be ultra-ultra sweet, addictive, and damaging to your brain. They can trigger a sweet-tooth attack.
- Chew some xylitol gum. Just be sure to avoid the fake sweeteners (as above) and corn syrup in most gums.
- Take a very hot shower. Don't burn yourself, but allow the water to be so hot that it's uncomfortable. Stand with your back to the water for 5–10 minutes.
- Hot saunas or steam rooms can have the same effect. You will feel more relaxed, and the craving will be gone.

- Avoid excess stress.
- Get enough sleep. A lack of sleep can increase cortisol levels, dysregulate your blood sugar, and feed your cravings.
- Avoid triggers like walking past ice cream parlors on your way to lunch.
- Avoid people who eat a lot of junk food and wave it in your face.
- Surround yourself with people who are supportive and who eat healthfully.
- Make sure your gut is healthy and that you're eating a wide variety of healthy vegetables, fats, and meats. If you aren't absorbing the nutrients from your food, then you may have nutritional deficiencies that could cause cravings. This includes parasitic infections that can impact cravings.
- Go cold turkey, and stay brave! Implement your willpower.

Emotional Craving

Craving sweets can also be viewed from an emotional and spiritual perspective. Are you craving sweeter experiences? Do you feel bitter toward people, situations, or events? If you have trouble finding any sweetness in your life, you may be using food as a substitute in an unhealthy way.

Unfortunately, giving in to a sweet craving will feed into the cycle of addiction, and your dissatisfaction with life will simply continue unaddressed. Ask yourself questions like, "Where do I already have sweetness in my life?" or "What relationships, creative expressions, or experiences sweeten my existence?" You can ask yourself, what is this craving showing you about yourself or any unmet needs? Then meet them for yourself in a healthy way.

A Carb-Craving Story

I had a patient called "Rosa." She felt and looked inflamed. She had regular vaginal discomfort and pain, plus digestive problems. She suffered from ADD and had trouble focusing and following through on tasks. She had strong sweet cravings and an addiction to corn. Rosa couldn't imagine life without corn chips and popcorn.

She had several strongly negative emotional reactions to my food recommendations—sure signs of imbalances. Rather than pushing those feelings away or judging them, I helped Rosa embrace and honor them in ways that left her feeling strong rather than beaten up. Then during a follow-up session, she reported feeling very "deprived."

A sense of deprivation is quite common and, fortunately, easy to shift. Rosa and I traced the origins of the deprived feeling, which ultimately were about a lack of affection and love in her life, not food. We processed the various layers of her feelings, beliefs, and experiences, harmonizing each piece we discovered.

The result? Once she understood she'd used food for comfort and gained tools to get her needs met in a healthier, more balanced way, she easily shifted away from her addictions to sugar and corn. She no longer wanted things that weren't nourishing. We fine-tuned her nutritional plan to make sure her brain and metabolism were functioning optimally. She lost weight, the puffy inflammation subsided, the vaginal discomfort calmed, and her digestion improved.

Craving Sugar Is a Symptom

There's no need to shame yourself; instead, explore the root causes and heal, so that you are free. Also remember that a craving is not the same as hunger. That said, if you allow yourself to become hungry on top of having a craving, it's most likely going to end up in disaster. Your will collapses, and you end up beating yourself up.

Commit to loving yourself enough to dig deep into your psyche and see where your life remains unfulfilling. Get support, and make changes. Love yourself enough to learn to override your cravings and eat something healthy, even if it doesn't seem very appetizing in the moment. Over time, the cravings should diminish, and you will be free—vibrantly healthy and happy, with much more energy. So, stay off the sweet stuff!

Part III

The Functional Ketogenic Gut Repair Program

Changing your diet and lifestyle can be scary and uncomfortable. I want to let you know I understand this. On top of that, our culture has molded us to resist pain and pursue pleasure.

But how much more painful is ill health, chronic physical pain, physical and mental impairment, and uncertainty? Surely a little short-term discomfort as you get on the healing path is a good trade against a lifetime of incapacitation?

There is more to this program than eliminating certain foods you may crave. There are emotional and psychological components to both ill health and healing. If the subject matter in this book brings up excuses, fear, disconnection (as in you check out), hostility, denial, paralysis, and any other strong emotional reaction, please realize that there's a juicy unresolved issue inside you showing up in order to be explored and for healing to occur.

Don't worry. I'm here to help empower you to love yourself enough to bring awareness and resolution to old issues so you can truly thrive. As we move forward in the Functional Ketogenic Gut Repair Program, I will address such things as feeling deprived and not knowing what to eat when you go out with friends. I won't leave you hanging!

Remember: True healing often needs us to lean into the emotional pain points a little in order to better understand, feel, and fully release them. And this is ultimately liberating.

Chapter 11

Becoming Ketogenic— Everything You Need

*K*etosis is a metabolic state characterized by raised ketone levels in the body tissues. *Ketones* are alternative fuel molecules your body makes in the liver from fat when glucose (blood sugar) levels are low. There are ways to induce this therapeutic state, which helps heal your gut, modulate your immune system, optimize brain function, and decrease inflammation.

Three main types of ketones are found in the body: acetone, acetoacetate, and beta-hydroxybutyrate. As you move into ketosis, your body will produce different types of ketones, in varying amounts. Methods to test your ketones include:

Blood Ketone Meter. This is the most accurate way of testing but also the priciest. It tests for beta-hydroxybutyrate (BHB), considered a ketone body. A meter may be about $40 and test strips $5 each, so it can add up during your first month. If you have the financial ability to invest in this method, it's very accurate.

Breathalyzer Test. This measures breath acetone concentration, a ketone body that results from the breakdown of acetoacetate. It's important to note that this test can be affected by alcohol consumption and dehydration. This test doesn't always correlate with blood ketones, but it is an inexpensive test.

Ketone Urine Strips. These are less accurate, because they only show excess ketone bodies that are excreted through the urine and don't tell you the level of BHB in your blood, which is likely much higher. As you become keto-adapted, your body will produce different ketones at varying levels.

Urine strips only measure acetoacetate, which may or may not become detectable. Your hydration also impacts this test—higher water intake will dilute the ketones in your urine. This test is inexpensive—about $10 for 50 strips.

Observe Your Body. This approach is free but requires awareness. You may notice your breath, sweat, or urine smelling like acetone. This is commonly referred to as "fruity" breath; in extreme cases of diabetic ketoacidosis, it can smell like nail polish remover. A fruity, acetone body odor, breath, or urine likely means you're in ketosis.

Note: If you choose to test yourself, be sure to check ketone levels three times per day when you're starting out: Morning, one hour after lunch, and before bed. You will also want to purchase a small notebook to record your readings and carbohydrate intake.

Three Ways to Achieve Ketosis

Here are three methods for reaching a state of ketosis:

Very Low Carb. Start with 15 grams of carbs a day and slowly decrease by 5 grams per day until ketones rise above 0.6 mmol. (Other doctors, nutritionists, and health coaches may recommend readings be closer to 1.5–3 mmol. I've found it depends on the patient, their lifestyle, genetics, health history, and metabolism.) This starts you out on a very low and restricted carbohydrate intake. Some people must keep carbohydrates below 20 grams in order to get into ketosis and remain there. Some people feel the impact of this; others don't. I believe it is the fastest way to get into ketosis, other than fasting, but you are more likely to experience the "ketoflu" if you go too fast. (See below).

Moderate Carb. If you're eating a lot of carbs, you can start with 60–75 grams of carbs per day and reduce by 5–10 grams per day until ketones rise above 0.6 mmol. This is a gentler way to ease off the carbohydrates; it may be the way to go if you're a heavy carb lover and want to take it easy. It will take longer to reach ketosis, but you may prefer the gradual transition. (I've included higher-carbohydrate recipes for this transitional period in the recipe section at the end of this book.)

Water Fast. The most extreme way to reach ketosis is through a water-only fast. The initial fast should last 12–72 hours and be followed by eating 75–90 percent healthy fat, 15–20 percent protein, and 5–10 percent nonstarchy carbohydrate in the form of leafy green vegetables per day. Most people I work with have blood sugar issues, so this is not for them unless they can take a few days off from work. **Note:** If you have low blood sugar, can't function well if you skip a meal or get crabby, or if you have polycystic ovarian syndrome (PCOS), then fasting may not be in your best interest.

If you reduce carbohydrates too quickly, don't increase your fat enough, and don't get enough micronutrients, your body can go into a starvation response and release cortisol stress hormones, which is your body's way of protecting your brain by raising your blood sugar levels. Do your best to create a peaceful environment and life during your nutritional changes. Taking adaptogenic herbs can help, as well as gradually restricting carbohydrates.

KETOGENIC TIP: Consider taking exogenous beta-hydroxybutyrate (BHB). It can quickly increase your measurable blood ketone level two-plus points, give you more energy quickly, and support your move into ketosis as well as maintain it. The manufacturers claim it increases athletic performance, and this has also been my experience.

Decreasing your carbohydrate intake is the first step in achieving ketosis. You must simultaneously increase your healthy fat intake and consume adequate quantities of raw sea salt. Your body needs salt when you are ketogenic. The mainstream food media has demonized salt, and even made you believe it will cause high blood pressure, but this isn't true. The general rule of thumb is about two teaspoons of raw salt a day. I prefer pink Himalayan sea salt or gray Celtic sea salt because they have more minerals in them. This can also decrease or eliminate possible ketoflu symptoms.

KETOGENIC TIP: Getting into ketosis usually requires strict carbohydrate restriction. Once ketosis is obtained you can add a little carb in the form of sweet potato or grain-free coconut bread and still remain in ketosis. Everyone is different. It's an art, so listen to your body, test if necessary, and enjoy extra energy, no hunger pains, balanced weight, better brain function, and so much more.

How to Test Your Blood Sugar

Check fasting glucose by testing 20 minutes after you wake up, or 12 hours after your last meal, with no snacks but drinking lots of water. When tracking your glucose, test two hours after each meal to see how your body is dealing with blood sugar levels. You may do this if you are prediabetic, have markers of possible future insulin resistance, or are currently insulin resistant. Blood sugar should be approximately 88–100 when testing several hours after a meal.

Healthy Fats

As you move toward ketosis, consuming healthy fats is essential. Avoid cooking with cottonseed, canola (rapeseed), safflower, sunflower, corn, and soy oils, as these kinds of vegetable oils are prone to harmful oxidation and rancidity and excess quantities cause inflammation. The process of making oil from seeds is difficult, requiring chemicals and heat. This causes the oil to become rancid long before you cook with it. It may not smell rancid, because it has been deodorized, which further strips it of any good omega-3 fats, but its anti-health properties remain.

Healthy fats for cooking and drizzling over your food include olive oil (never subject it to heat), coconut oil, avocado oil, duck fat, beef fat, grapeseed oil, and red palm oil (please purchase environmentally friendly brands due to the destruction of orangutan habitat). All should be organic. Nut oils, such as Brazil nut oil, pepita or pumpkin seed oil, and macadamia nut oil, should not be heated. Depending on your gut repair program, avoid nut oils for the first two months, then you may incorporate them and see how you feel.

Side Effects of a Ketogenic Nutritional Plan

The side effects of becoming ketogenic are minimal. Some of the first signs of moving into healthy ketosis are known as the "keto flu". For a short time, you may experience symptoms like headache, increased hunger, brain fog, fatigue, decreased performance when you exercise, crabbiness, sleep issues, and nausea. These symptoms are more likely to appear if you're moving too quickly into ketosis and your electrolyte balance is off. Read on how to treat and avoid these symptoms. These will subside within two to five days on average. If you can tolerate temporary, minor symptoms, your body will thank you.

If you have candida, fungal infections, parasites, or other bacteria present in your body or gut, you may have a detoxifying reaction. It would then be best to eliminate carbohydrates more slowly, adopting my second proposed way to move into ketosis and test ketones by beginning with 60–75 grams of carbohydrates a day and then decreasing by 5–10 grams per day until you reach ketosis.

Do this with professional support. There are many variables, and you are an individual. It is important that you work with someone who knows your unique set of circumstances.

Tips to Help with "Keto Flu" Symptoms

- Drink plenty of spring water (not reverse osmosis). Calculate your body weight in pounds, divide by two, and add 16 ounces more to that number. This will give you the number of ounces of water you need daily. (The metric calculation: divide your weight in kg by 30, then add 0.5, and that is the number of liters you need daily.)
- If you exercise and live in the desert or a hot climate, add another 8–16 ounces or 250–500 ml. It's generally a good rule to approximate 1 gallon or 3.8 l per day per person; this amount includes water used for cooking and so forth.
- The functional ketogenic gut repair plan has a diuretic effect, so keeping your electrolytes balanced is important. You may notice you pee more. Begin adding high-grade, unrefined sea salt to your diet. You may also consider adding liquid trace minerals, following the dose on the bottle and increasing gradually to an optimal dose. Or you can supplement with 3,000–4,000 mg sodium, 1,000 mg potassium, and 300 mg magnesium. Look for commercially available single liquid minerals, marine minerals, or liquid trace minerals.
- When you're crabby, or "hangry," reach for healthy fats.
- Some people need to increase their fat intake more slowly for proper digestion. I use ox bile, enzymes, betaine HCl, bitters, and pepsin to support digesting increased fat intake while maintaining a healthy gallbladder.
- Get plenty of sleep.
- Move your body (if symptoms aren't too bothersome). Exercise can really help.
- Get out in nature.
- Watch a good comedy and laugh. Laughter can help both your mind and body.
- Your metabolism is transforming. Take a nap and allow your body to process the changes. It's important to sleep well at night, and it's okay to rest during the first few days if you aren't feeling well.

- Get support by connecting with others who will build up your confidence to keep going.

Is It Safe to Remain on a Ketogenic Diet for a Long Period of Time?

Yes, it is. One study analyzed a 24-week ketogenic program and concluded that there are no harmful side effects and several beneficial effects to being on a long-term ketogenic diet, including reduced body weight and body mass index; decreased levels of triglycerides, LDL (bad) cholesterol, and blood glucose; along with an increase in the level of HDL (good) cholesterol.

KETOGENIC TIP: Going ketogenic, your metabolism and body are going to undergo a fabulous transformation and some people have cravings or feel hungry in the beginning. When you're hungry or craving something, reach for fat, salt, and water. Eating healthy fats like an avocado or coconut butter, adding sea salt, and drinking lots of spring water will help immediately.

When Is Ketogenic Gut Repair Complete?

Several markers indicate when intensive gut repair is complete and you are ready to move to the maintenance phase. First is the complete resolution of your symptoms. The pitfall to watch out for is that you can feel totally better and still have gut damage that will provoke more symptoms over time. This is why I rely on both indicators, the alleviation of symptoms backed by comprehensive testing.

Gut repair can take six months. In the meantime, it's necessary to avoid foods that cause inflammation, including hidden food sensitivities, stress, toxins, and poor lifestyle choices. This may seem impossible. But what it boils down to is doing your best and managing the things over which you have control, trusting that your body will heal and detoxify in the face of your good choices.

You'll always face exposure to chemicals, stress, and foods you aren't aware cause inflammation. However, with a healed, healthy gut, your body is more likely to handle these challenges with ease.

KETOGENIC GUT REPAIR PLAN TIPS

- After you are ketogenic, you can begin to have small amounts of higher-carb foods, such as sweet potato (½–1 cup or 120–240 ml), parsnip soup, butternut squash, and so on. But it's best to have these in the evening. Do your best to consume lower-carb veggies, such as leafy greens, during the day. If, in the beginning of your ketogenic plan, you're craving sweets and you're crabby and irritable, it's okay to introduce a tiny bit of carb into your evening meal.
- Exercise! Try exercising in the morning during your fasting time. This is also ideal for your cortisol levels. I've found that exercise curbs my appetite when I'm ketogenic or on my way to it. There's a fine line with this. If I exercise too much, my appetite increases; if I do moderate, high-intensity interval training (HIIT), it curbs my appetite. You'll find your own sweet spot.
- Avoid eating higher-carbohydrate foods with lots of fat. Carbohydrates cause your insulin to spike. If this happens in the presence of fat, you're hurting yourself more than helping. The fat and carbs will be stored and not burned as fuel.
- For some people, eating a very high-protein diet can prevent them from staying in ketosis. Eating around 0.5 g protein/lb lean body weight seems a good rule of thumb. You can make ATP (energy) by converting protein and amino acids via a process called *gluconeogenesis*. Your body will only convert what it needs while still making ketone bodies. I haven't found evidence that moderate protein will throw you out of ketosis.
- Get to know your body better! Begin to differentiate feeling full versus feeling satisfied. In our society, there's a huge rise in emotional eating and diagnosable eating disorders. We often eat for comfort. Begin to notice if you're satisfied both physically and emotionally by the food you eat.
- Are you really hungry or just craving something? If you're craving sugar or starches, reach for healthy fats. If you 're really hungry, eat fat, protein, and vegetables.

- Alcohol can cause your insulin levels to spike, which knocks down your ketones. It's better to have alcohol with food to minimize insulin spikes and drops in ketones. The ideal is to eliminate it.
- Your environment affects your ability to remain in ketosis. Lack of sleep, stress, trauma, infections, and toxic exposures may throw you out of ketosis.
- If you've done a low-carb nutritional plan before and "it didn't work," then it's likely there were other issues that need to be addressed. You may have hypothyroidism, insulin resistance, diabetes, latent infection, adrenal fatigue, or hormone imbalances that weren't properly addressed. You may have had the wrong proportions of fat, protein, and vegetables. Don't give up. Instead, give it your all. You're an individual and need to find what works for you. Get support.
- Anything that raises insulin levels in your body can throw you out of ketosis. Sometimes hormones are the culprit. In this case, liver support is very important.
- You don't need to limit caloric intake. Instead, watch foods that increase insulin.
- Focus on lowering carbs, increasing healthy fats, and not increasing your protein. Unless you are a vegetarian or vegan most Americans get plenty of protein.

A Note on Fasting

Intermittent fasting (14–16 hours) is very supportive to staying in ketosis but not always necessary. I prefer to do part of my fasting in my sleep and then the rest in the morning. I've encountered many people who have blood sugar stabilization issues, which usually clear up if they are in ketosis long enough. Fasting may or may not be beneficial for your body and metabolic type in the beginning. Once you are ketogenic, then fasting is much easier, without side effects like headaches and blood sugar crash fatigue.

KETOGENIC TIP: Fasting for my keto gut repair plan means no chewing of food, but drinking is okay. I recommend ½ to a full can of full-fat coconut milk with a scoop of toasted maca powder, a dash of cinnamon, raw vanilla powder, a scoop of protein powder (see section "A Word on Protein Powders" on page 100), and green grass powders. Once you've done two months of gut repair, you can add a heaping scoop of raw cacao or toasted carob powder. All of these ingredients are optional. The full-fat coconut milk is the kind of fat you need to help you get into and remain in ketosis.

THE SCIENCE
FASTING AND STEM CELLS

Fasting isn't all bad. It can help your stem cell production, which helps your tissue regenerate! One study (Cheng et al., 2014) found that fasting can actually promote regulating hematopoietic stem cell protection, self-renewal, and regeneration. This study found that the immunosuppression as well as cell death caused by chemotherapy was diminished by multiple cycles of fasting. Lymphocytes were protected from chemotoxicity in fasting patients. Prolonged fasting also reduces circulating IGF-1 levels and PKA activity in various cell populations.[85]

Chapter 12
Functional Testing

Proper testing is a highly recommended part of my Functional Ketogenic Gut Repair Program. In today's Western medical world, we operate under a "sick care" or "disease-management" model. Functional, holistic, and comprehensive healthcare focuses on education, early detection, prevention, and individualized treatment of both symptoms and root causes. Ideally, it also honors cultural, lifestyle, and emotional factors, thus empowering people toward optimum health and well-being.

Conventional blood chemistry analysis (the interpretation of blood work) determines what is normal according to ranges compiled from a tiny sampling of patients, most of whom are having their blood analyzed because they're already ill—often severely ill. Or standards are set from recommendations in books or packaging inserts. But when a patient's blood falls within the range of "normal" among a group of sick people, can that accurately say anything about their wellness? No!

You could call this "dysfunctional blood chemistry analysis." By contrast, functional blood chemistry analysis (FBCA) compiles its ranges based on health, wellness, and optimal functioning.

Functionally normal ranges are much narrower than their conventional dysfunctional counterparts. When a person's levels fall within functionally normal ranges, we can be much more confident about the health of the bodily system measured by that blood component. When a person's levels fall outside functional ranges but remain within conventional ranges, we can consider it a red flag of imbalance, possibly indicating disease patterns that conventional medicine may not recognize (sub-clinical). By catching imbalances before tissues are damaged and symptoms manifest, your health outlook is greatly improved.

FBCA is an effective and efficient tool for identifying imbalances in the body's metabolism. Bottom line, there is no general screening test that is more efficient, effective, and affordable than a comprehensive functional blood chemistry panel.

But a comprehensive panel must be ordered. I like to see close to 70 markers, plus a urinalysis. This includes a full thyroid panel of eight markers of thyroid function, plus two thyroid antibody tests. I haven't met an endocrinologist yet who orders a comprehensive thyroid panel, but they quickly rush to give a patient T4 (thyroid) drug therapy for an elevated thyroid-stimulating hormone (TSH), failing to actually identify the root of the imbalance or discover if T4 is even the correct drug to use. I don't mean to put down doctors. They're doing their very best with the tools and training they have. It just often isn't good enough. And I want the best for you!

So, why doesn't your doctor want to test you more thoroughly?

First, few Western-trained medical doctors and naturopaths are versed in FBCA, nor do they know how to order appropriate comprehensive panels. The second reason is there's a "standard of care" in the US that MDs must follow or lose their license. This standard of care dictates what they must do with your test results. For example, if you're having gout symptoms and your uric acid is high, an indicator of possible gout, insulin resistance/diabetes, oxidative stress or kidney issues, then the standard of care requires them to prescribe a drug to bring it down, most commonly in the form of a xanthine oxidase inhibitor, such as allopurinol or colchicine for pain.

The standard of care doesn't acknowledge the question of why the uric acid is high or why the symptoms of gout appeared, and it doesn't require further investigation to determine the answer; instead, it requires instant medication. And yet gout is often easily treated with a few nutritional and lifestyle shifts and one or two supplements!

Finding the root cause of your symptoms is not part of the current healthcare model, so your doctor won't order the right tests. If they do order tests outside the standard of care, often they don't know how to interpret them properly. They aren't trained to find the why; they're only trained to medicate the symptoms. This is a real bummer if you have thyroid challenges, gut issues, or any tricky health problem. In my experience, people with thyroid dysfunction, gut issues, and many other disease patterns are being seriously mismanaged in the current healthcare model.

I admit, I get frustrated when I think of all the people who are taking thyroid medication even though no doctor has ever fully evaluated a comprehensive lab panel, including a full thyroid panel with all 10 markers. (Technically, there are 11 markers, but that last one is only used for people with suspected Grave's disease.) The "gold standard" thyroid test is TSH, which is a hormone actually secreted by your pituitary gland. It measures if your pituitary is working, but not if your thyroid hormones are functioning properly. This seems crazy to me. Often TSH may be normal while other things are out of balance with your thyroid, but you won't ever know what's really going on if you don't test the right things.

FBCA enables healthcare practitioners to more effectively assist people with proper nutrition, supplementation, lifestyle, and treatment plans to better meet their health needs. It leads to selection of the most appropriate follow-up diagnostic tools and referrals to specialists. In my own journey to healing, FBCA has been a lifesaver. After years of misdiagnosis, comprehensive testing and functional interpretation of my lab results finally opened up a whole new world of understanding about what my body was trying to tell me and how best to support its movement toward health. I'm forever grateful for the wise pioneers in this field who are making these tools available!

Beyond FBCA, specific gut and food tests are important so that you can individualize your Functional Ketogenic Gut Repair Plan. The gut is definitely "hidden territory." Although you can usually tell what state your gut is in from external indicators already listed, figuring out what to actually do about it can be a guessing game.

For example, thousands of people realize that they're sensitive to gluten, or have actually been diagnosed with celiac disease and are doing their best to avoid foods that contain gluten; yet, their efforts are often insufficient, and they keep suffering—which is incredibly disheartening.

Why does this happen?

The trouble is, many foods that ought not to contain gluten actually contain trace amounts due to cross-contamination during processing. Even small amounts of inflammatory foods, such as grains, gluten, and dairy, can create an immune reaction in your intestinal membranes and body that can last for days, weeks, or even months. The second problem is gluten-associated cross-reactive foods, which do not contain gluten but have proteins with similar structure (antigenic similarity) to the gliadin protein found in gluten.

Your body may produce antibodies to a single gluten antigen or a combination of gluten antigens that may be cross-reactive with other food antigens. In the case of celiac disease, small amounts of non-gluten active proteins in the diet, such as the protein called avenin (from oats), can prevent healing of the intestinal tract mucosal lining.

A lot of people try to determine which foods they need to avoid by conducting their own food elimination test—trying a food and seeing if they react, then eliminating it from their diet. The trouble with this approach is someone with IgA food sensitivity may not have a reaction for a week after eating the food. In fact, IgG food sensitivity reaction may be delayed for up to a *month*. Which means people doing this on their own don't stand a chance of figuring out the source of their headache, itchy eyes, PMS, or constipation when they occur weeks later. This is why I call them hidden food sensitivities.

Another example of the need for specialized testing is people who have autoimmune tendencies. There are approximately 80 named autoimmune disorders, and many have similar general symptoms, such as fatigue, joint ache, brain fog, inflammation, low-grade fever, and an overall unwell feeling. Most people are diagnosed only *after* organ systems have sustained enough damage to show specific symptoms—including blood tests markers well outside clinical lab ranges (if tests are ever even done). If the state of autoimmunity can be identified *prior* to tissue damage, symptoms, and conventional clinical lab imbalances, the disease process can be halted and often reversed. Running accurate lab tests is the only way to realistically do this, and a test offered by Cyrex labs called Array 5 Multiple Autoimmune Reactivity Screening can show predictive antibodies. See below for details.

Recommended Functional Tests
Cyrex Labs Array 10, the Multiple Food Immune Reactivity Screen
This test evaluates immune reactions to foods (raw and/or cooked), food enzymes, lectins, herbs, spices, and food additives, including meat glue, artificial colorings, and gums. It is excellent for early detection of dietary-related triggers of autoimmune reactivity. It tests both raw and cooked foods. (Many people will react to one food raw but not cooked, or vice versa.) Eat the foods on the panel for 7 days in a row and then wait 26 days to be tested in order to get reliable results. If you react to any of these foods, it's recommended to avoid them for 4–6 months and then retest. While you are avoiding the foods, carrying out a comprehensive gut repair program will likely support you to eat most of the foods again, although there may be some that you must avoid eating forever.

This test shines a light on two aspects of your immune system and how it views foods by identifying hidden food sensitivities. Some foods, even healthy ones, such as vegetables, fruits, nuts, and meat, may be viewed by your body as a foreign invader. Your immune system may misidentify certain foods as viruses or bacteria in need of destruction. This test is quite valuable and can help clear up a few if not many of your health mysteries.

I urge you to investigate how your gut and immune system are really performing and discover which foods or combinations of foods trigger negative reactions. Find out whether you have predictive antibodies correlated with any major organs or tissues in your body. Accurate diagnostic information, coupled with excellent nutrition and inner work through the mind–body–spirit connection, is the key to prevention and treatment of all health challenges.

A TEST CASE
MY OWN

I'd had spastic bladder symptoms on and off since college. I'd often get a burning sensation in my urethra, had urgent and frequent urination, and pain. If I was the tiniest bit dehydrated, or rode my road bike too long, or held my urine during a car trip, or any combination of these with sex, BOOM! I'd have painful symptoms. Dip sticks and urine cultures would usually test negative for bacteria indicating bladder infections—which I sometimes got as well.

It was a bummer and really disrupted my life until a urologist finally diagnosed me. I didn't love the idea of taking medications that had pages of side effects, but at least he gave me a list of foods to avoid, which I did. From trial and error I discovered that wine, kombucha, and almonds instantly triggered my symptoms, but it turned out that there were more hidden ones as well. It was only after I had trusted and hidden food sensitivities tested, IgG and IgA tests done, that I solved the mystery.

I had four food sensitivities to vegetables, fruits, and one fish that I'd considered quite healthy and had been eating at least weekly. When I omitted these foods from my diet, the spastic bladder symptoms stopped completely.

Cyrex Labs Array 2 Intestinal Antigenic Permeability Screen
This test measures the gut's capacity to absorb nutrients, the degree to which it allows non-nutrients to pass into the blood, the degree of accumulated tissue damage, and the ratio of healthy/unhealthy bacterial flora. It tests for intestinal antigenic permeability (leaky gut), dysbiosis (unhealthy

flora), epithelial cell damage, and tight junction damage, providing a solid baseline for all people tested—especially those with any digestive, skin, immune, neurological, or emotional challenges. The test can be repeated to measure progress in healing all types of gut challenges and auto-immunity, including celiac disease.

Cyrex Labs Array 11 Chemical Immune Reactivity Test

This test measures predictive antibodies to a variety of antigens, such as chemicals, pesticides, metals, and so on, and should always be considered to detect any body burden patterns. The chemicals being measured in this test are those that can often contribute to gut damage and inflammation.

Cyrex Labs Array 4 Gluten-Associated Cross-Reactive Foods and Foods Sensitivity

This tests for common primary-reactive foods, such as coffee, sesame, buckwheat, sorghum, hemp, amaranth, quinoa, tapioca, teff, soy, egg, and potato, plus common cross-reactive foods, such as rye, barley, spelt, wheat, milk products (casein, casomorphin, butyrophilin, whey, milk chocolate), oats, yeast, millet, corn, and rice. Often, people new to a gluten-free diet over-consume common starchy foods or are introduced to new foods that elicit cross-reaction. Their symptoms may not shift or easily return because of these other, unidentified, cross-reactive foods.

Array 4 can help determine what is best for your body. You must eat all the foods on the list for at least seven days in a row. Then you wait 26 days for your blood draw. This gives your body time to make antibodies to the food antigens to which you cross-react.

Note: If you have celiac or know you are sensitive to any food on the panel, especially gluten, I would dissuade you from consuming it. It's not worth eating gluten for the test, especially if you know you react. Simply avoid this food for life, and rest assured you're taking great care of your health and future. Yes, that's right. I said *for life*. You may feel shocked that I suggest this, and it can seem extreme at first, but if you cross-react or have a strong sensitivity to a food you may need to avoid it forever in order to remain well and symptom-free.

Cyrex Labs Array 5 Multiple Autoimmune Reactivity Screen

The development of an autoimmune disease may be influenced by a triad of factors: genetic vulnerability, immune system response to environ-mental exposures (toxic chemicals, antigenic foods, infectious agents), and intestinal permeability. A predictive antibody test is a vital tool in the prevention and treatment of autoimmune disorders. This test measures even low-level antibodies to almost every vital organ, tissue, and gland, including IgG and IgA, combined of the following: adrenal cortex, cerebellum, insulin and islet cell antigen associated with diabetes, myelin basic protein, phospholipid, intrinsic factor, parietal cells, myocardial peptide, arthritic peptide, osteocyte, collagen complex, synapsin, and many more.

A trained functional healthcare practitioner can provide lifesaving information that will keep you healthy and happy.

If immune dysfunction is suspected, clues can be found in family history, including cancer, rheumatoid arthritis, multiple sclerosis, lupus, diabetes, thyroid dysfunction, cancer, or intestinal trouble such as irritable bowel syndrome or Crohn's disease. It is well known that if one autoimmune disease is present, it's likely that another will develop. This test can tell you which organs, tissues, and glands are targeted so that you can halt the attack and protect your organs before irreversible damage has occurred. The Array 5 test can also help track antibody levels and identify preventative measures. This insight is essential for fine-tuning your nutritional and lifestyle program.

Also, comprehensive stool and urine analyses can identify other areas of digestive and gut health. Some labs are better than others in how effectively their equipment detects parasites or other imbalances. Please consult a holistic, functional, and integrative healthcare provider.

A Final Word on Testing

If you seek testing, understand that when you retest stool or blood, you'll see specific changes. For example, if you do Cyrex Array 2, you'll note improvements across the board. You must consult with a holistic healthcare provider in order to properly interpret these results. When accurately reading a comprehensive lab panel, you will also note that specific markers of digestion improve. Again, this requires a trained holistic and functional healthcare provider who is well versed in reading labs according to *functional reference ranges* to understand their meanings. My next book, *Know Your Blood, Know Your Health*, will empower you around functional blood chemistry analysis in detail.

Finding the right professional support can give you what you need to heal. If one practitioner doesn't work out, don't give up. When you find the right people, get the right tests (now that you know what they are!), and obtain the critical health information that applies only to *you*, then you can and will heal.

Chapter 13

Food: The Foundation of Keto Gut Repair

I know this is the chapter you've been waiting for. What can I eat? What can't I eat? That's the question! You already know the main points of the Functional Ketogenic Gut Repair Plan: low in carbohydrates (1 ounce or 30 g or less per day), lots of healthy fats, moderate amounts of protein (2–4 ounces or 60–120 g twice per day), ZERO grains and starchy vegetables but HIGH in other veggies. Let's get to the details.

The good news is that you should never be hungry. You can eat regular meals and snack throughout the day—there is no caloric restriction. The goal of this nutritional plan is to eliminate dietary triggers that cause intestinal inflammation so that your body can repair itself, self-modulate immune function, and prevent, mediate, or halt health challenges, such as autoimmune issues.

I know that changing your relationship with food, your body, and your health is a huge step. But I'm here to help walk you through it, step by step—baby steps or giant steps, it's up to you to decide what works for you. Connecting with your fears and resistance is an important part of this program. Please don't suppress these emotions or actions, which may be sabotaging your healing, health, and even your relationships. Rather, I invite you to dive more deeply into them, investigating their origins. I offer contemplative exercises in Chapter 16 that will help.

It's important to closely adhere to the nutrition and lifestyle gut-repair plan in this book in order to stop your body's self-reinforcing cycle of *dysbiosis* (microbial imbalance), malabsorption of nutrients, and permeability to non-nutrients. If you have autoimmunity or a diagnosed autoimmune disease, or other chronic gut issues like irritable bowel disease, then the stricter you are, the more likely you are to halt the disease process and prevent future autoimmune flare-ups. Ultimately, this means far less suffering. Remember that an unhealthy gut develops over time—which means repairing it will also take time.

Many people who need gut repair also have dysbiosis caused by an overgrowth of yeast (often referred to as candida). Therefore, it's best to avoid all fruits, which feed the yeast. Low-glycemic fruits such as berries are allowed only if you have stable blood sugar and you've been tested for gut permeability and candida. Otherwise, it may be best to avoid all fruit for the first two to four months and then slowly reintroduce berries into the plan, depending on how long you wish to be ketogenic.

If there are foods on the plan that don't work for you because they cause pain, gas, bloating, energy crashes, or skin problems, or you've tested positive for IgE, IgG, IgA, or other sensitivities to those foods—omit them.

TIPS AND TRICKS

Going out to dinner. Order grilled salmon or chicken without sauces, with a side order of stir-fried or steamed veggies or a spinach salad. Drizzle olive oil on the meat and salad at the table, and add salt. Ask for rosemary with the chicken or dill and lemon with salmon. Remember KISS (Keep It Simple, Sweetie).

Be aware in Thai restaurants. Often commercial cans of coconut milk have wheat or gluten as a thickener. Ask to read the ingredients, just to be safe.

Watch for cross-contamination. Especially if you have celiac or find you have cross-reactivity via Cyrex Array 4 testing. If you are at a hamburger place, ask if they use a separate grill for the buns or if they use another side of the grill.

When traveling. Bring snacks in case of delays or cancellations. You'll be grateful to have some stir-fry, meat, or beef jerky on hand.

At parties. Take a dish you love and can share, so you know there will be food you can eat. Have potlucks and offer scrumptious recipes from this book. This is a fun way to teach friends about your new way of cooking and how delicious it can be.

As you follow the plan, remember that food is not the only source of inflammation. Lifestyle, medication, infections, poor sleep, and unresolved emotions can also cause inflammation and this perpetuates the cycle of declining gut health by damaging the intestinal mucosa.

Important: I highly recommend following this plan as strictly as humanly possible. But you know yourself. If you're not quite able to be that strict with yourself, don't worry. You can still gain tons of benefit by following this nutritional and lifestyle plan closely. Even if you desire slightly higher carbs than my Functional Ketogenic Gut Repair Plan includes, you can still gain healing. Don't sabotage yourself by quitting because you're not following the plan "perfectly." But also know if you don't get the results you desire, you may want to explore any resistance you may have that could be sabotaging your success.

I've offered a scientifically based approach, and you can customize it to fit your lifestyle and individual nutritional needs. I've listed what I've found to be optimal, and you can implement any portion of this plan and still experience some degree of healing. You will be pleasantly surprised by how great you feel.

The Importance of Organic

Health food stores; co-ops; community-supported agriculture (CSA) groups, gardens, and farms; and farmers markets all carry organic produce, organic meats and poultry, organic cheeses, butter, and oils. Costco, Safeway, Fred Meyer, and other major chain grocery stores carry organic products as well.

And no wonder. Organic is the hottest, fastest-growing market in the entire food industry because people are catching on. They're waking up to just how badly our food has been poisoned with pesticides and herbicides and how much our soils have been depleted of minerals and other healthy micro-organisms. After watching the 2012 documentary film *Genetic Roulette: The Gamble of Our Lives* about the dangers of genetically modified organisms (GMOs) in agriculture, there was no turning back for me.

There's ample scientific evidence to prove that organically grown produce is more nutritious than conventionally grown produce. For example, a study published in 2010 by Washington State University found that organic strawberries had a "longer shelf life, greater dry matter, and higher antioxidant activity and concentrations of ascorbic acid and phenolic compounds" than their conventional counterparts."[86] The

Haughley Experiment was one of the largest studies done on organic food. They found that cows living on organic farms, fed organic produce, ate less but consistently produced more milk.[87] Organic really is better. If you need more proof, there is a whole world of scientific literature on the internet on this subject.

A Word on Protein Powders

Buyer beware, there are many protein powders out there. Avoid whey due to lactose content. Whey protein isolate has less lactose but still is not completely clean. Look for organic pea protein, a bovine albumin concentrate, a bone broth protein isolate, beef or chicken collagen hydrolysate, or grass-fed beef protein isolate with no added fillers or garbage. Protein powders that have additions of green powders, curcumin, boswellia, CoQ10, and alpha lipoic acid could be an excellent anti-inflammatory start. Some are sweetened with stevia or monk fruit and may contain MCT oil or coconut flour.

WHAT TO EAT

In order to thrive, your body needs daily micro-doses of thousands of different synergistically complementary phyto (plant-based) nutrients. Phytochemicals protect the plant from being attacked by insects and harmful UV radiation. They also protect us! Different categories of phyto-nutrients give us different benefits, so consuming a wide array of them is important.

A simple yet effective way to gauge the breadth of your phytonutrient intake is to assess the variety of colors in the fruits and vegetables you eat. You want to consume the greatest variety of colors you can. The greater the variety of phytonutrients, the more raw materials the body has to repair tissue, balance hormones and brain chemistry, maintain healthy immune function, decrease inflammation, repair DNA, and promote healthy cardio-vascular functioning.

Some doctors believe patients should avoid all root vegetables, such as carrots, beets, and parsnips, because they are high in starches and sugar. I agree with them in certain situations, but it depends on your constitution, level of gut dysbiosis and candida overgrowth, metabolism, adrenal health, patterns of imbalance, level of commitment to your health, willpower, and open mind/heartedness. Many people do just fine with very small amounts of these veggies. Others with insulin resistance, for example, may not.

Consult your healthcare provider to see what is best for your body and health goals. It's ideal to rotate your foods as much as possible and avoid eating the exact same thing each day. It's okay to make large batches and spread them out over a week. But the following week use different vegetables. This will help eliminate any potential for increasing food sensitivities, which can happen when you have gut issues and eat too much of the same thing too often.

Vegetables

Artichoke
Asparagus
Beets
Bok choy
Broccoli
Burdock root
Cabbage
Carrot
Cauliflower
Celery
Celery root
Chard
Chives
Collard greens
Cucumber
Dandelion greens
Fennel (anise)
Garlic
Kale
Kohlrabi (in moderation—no more than one per week; best to avoid for first two months)
Leeks
Lettuce (the deeper green or red, the better)
Mustard greens
Onions
Parsley
Parsnip

Radish
Rhubarb
Rutabaga/Swede
Shallots
Spinach
Sprouts
Sorrel (wonderful, slightly sour green, great in salads)
Squash (winter squash, such as butternut, acorn, and spaghetti and summer squash, such as yellow crookneck and zucchini/courgette). In moderation—no more than one per week; I recommend none for the first two months.
Sweet potatoes (in moderation—no more than ½–1 cup/120–240 ml per week; I recommend none for the first two months)
Water chestnuts
Watercress (a slightly spicy green also great in salads)
Yams (in moderation—no more than ½–1 cup/120–240 ml per week; I recommend none for the first two months)

Fermented Foods

Fermented foods are great for the gut, but avoid them if you have high histamine, histamine reactions, or candida issues. Some people do not do well with fermented drinks and foods. If you don't feel well, begin craving sugar, get bloated, or have bad breath from them, discontinue.

Kimchi	Sauerkraut (raw)
Kombucha tea	Unsweetened coconut yogurt
Pickled ginger (minus food coloring, MSG, and preservatives)	Unsweetened coconut kefir

Meats

The ideal meat is the one you've hunted yourself. (I'm not kidding. It's in alignment with our Paleolithic ancestors and is a highly spiritual process as well as a practical one.) Yes, I know that's probably not going to happen. Next best is wild meat. If you aren't a hunter, ask around and see if there are any in your community from whom you can buy. Your body will appreciate it! Next best is free-range buffalo, elk, lamb, rabbit, and other organic meats you can find at some butcher shops. Other than that, do your best to purchase organic, free-range, hormone-free, antibiotic-free, and pastured (grass-fed) animals that have not depended on corn and grains for their nutrients. **Note:** Don't get lean meat from the butcher. On a functional ketogenic plan, you want the fattier meats.

Beef	Lamb
Buffalo	Ostrich
Chicken	Pheasant
Dove	Quail
Elk	Rabbit
Kangaroo	Turkey

Wild-Caught Fish

Consume only minimal amounts of fish from the Pacific due to radiation poisoning. Consume larger fish, such as cod and tuna, in moderation. Avoid farmed fish, as they're fed unnatural food, have added food coloring, and swim in their own waste.

Anchovies	Salmon
Bass	Sardines
Cod	Red snapper
Halibut	Trout

Fruits

Always acceptable

Lemons

Limes

Avocados

Cucumbers

Reintroduce gradually

Speak with your healthcare provider to determine whether you will be fruit-free for the first two months, after which time you may begin to introduce the fruits listed below. If you're transitioning gradually, you may include berries, but in small quantities.

Berries, such as blueberries, raspberries, blackberries, strawberries, and açai

Cherries

Pomegranates

Cranberries

Goji berries (they are a nightshade but are loaded with nutritional and health benefits)

Reintroduce in moderation

These next fruits in moderation, and only after at least 2–4 months of intensive gut repair, or incorporate later if you don't wish to remain ketogenic:

Apples

Peaches

Pears

Apricots

Grapefruit

Plums

Coconut

Coconut butter is a staple in our home. Try it on baked veggies or root veggies! Cook with coconut oil, and remember to rotate your cooking oils. Use coconut cream, unsweetened coconut flakes, and unsweetened coconut yogurt. Raw, live, aged coconut with the brown husk is a crunchy lifesaver! See the Snack and Travel Food section for directions on cracking.

Oils

Unrefined is always best.

Avocado (great alternative to coconut oil for cooking)

Brazil nut oil (only use uncooked; hold off for first two months of gut repair)

Coconut oil (you can find refined, which is flavorless)

Duck/goose fat (great for cooking; stores well in the fridge)

Ghee (only ghee that is casein- and lactose-free)

Grapeseed oil (great alternative to coconut oil for cooking/ baking)

Macadamia nut oil (only use uncooked; hold off for first two months of gut repair)
Olive oil (only use uncooked)

Pumpkin (pepita) seed oil (only use uncooked; hold off for first two months of gut repair)
Walnut oil (only use uncooked; hold off for first two months of gut repair)

Herbs and Spices

Basil
Black pepper (avoid for first two months; it can be hard on the gut)
Borage
Cilantro (coriander leaves/stalks)
Coriander
Cumin
Curry
Dill
Garlic
Gynostemma (my favorite sugar-craving curb)
Ginger
Horsetail
Lemongrass
Maca leaf (different from root)

Maca root (often raw—gently toast it in a pan on the stove top to help release the adaptogenic healing properties)
Mint
Oregano
Parsley
Rosemary
Rose hips
Rose petals
Sage
Savory
Sea salt (raw—I prefer Celtic, which is gray with flecks, or pink Himalayan)
Tarragon
Thyme
Turmeric

Sweeteners

Monk fruit

Stevia

Other

Apple cider vinegar
Chia seeds (avoid if you have ulcerative colitis)

Flax seeds (avoid if you have ulcerative colitis)
Herbal teas (Tulsi, or holy basil)
Olives

FOODS TO AVOID

Sugars (natural and artificial sweeteners)

Agave	Honey
Coconut sugar	Maple syrup
Coconut syrup	Molasses
Corn syrup	Nutrasweet
Equal	Sucrose
Fructose	Sucralose
High-fructose corn syrup	Splenda

High-Glycemic Fruits

Bananas	Mango
Canned fruits	Papaya
Cantaloupe melon	Pineapple
Dried fruits, including	Raisins
cranberries	Watermelon

Nuts and Seeds

Almonds	Pecans
Brazil nuts	Pepitas
Flax seeds	Sunflower seeds
Hemp seeds	Sesame seeds
Macadamia nuts	Walnuts
Peanuts	

Grains

Amaranth	Oats
Barley	Quinoa
Buckwheat	Rice
Bulgur wheat	Rye
Corn	Semolina
Couscous	Spelt
Polished wheat	Wheat
Millet	Wheat germ

Gluten

You'll be amazed at how gluten seems to find its way into everything:

Barbecue sauces

Binders

Bouillon

Brewer's yeast

Condiments

Emulsifiers

Fillers

Gum

Hydrolyzed plant and
vegetable protein

Ketchup

Lunch meats

Malt and malt flavoring

Maltodextrin (can also be from
barley, rice, corn, and tapioca)

Malt vinegar

Matzo

Modified food starch

Monosodium glutamate (MSG)

Nondairy creamer

Processed meats (cold cuts,
hot dogs, sausages)

Processed salad dressings

Seitan

Some spice mixtures

Soy sauce

Stabilizers

Teriyaki sauce

Textured vegetable protein

Dairy

Eggs—They don't come from
cows, of course, but they're in
the dairy section and are a high
allergen for many!

Cow's milk

Goat's milk

Sheep's milk

Butter (ghee that is both
casein- and lactose-free is safe)

Cheese

Cream

Frozen desserts

Margarine

Mayonnaise

Whey

Yogurt (except for
unsweetened coconut or
almond)

Soy

Edamame

Miso (can find it made from
legumes, which is better)

Soy milk

Soy protein

Soy sauce

Tempeh

Tofu

Fungi

Mushrooms

Edible fungi

Alcohol

All alcohol

Beans and Legumes

Adzuki beans

Black beans

Kidney beans

Lentils

Mung beans

Peanuts

Pinto beans

Soybeans

White beans

Nightshades

Eggplant

Paprika

Peppers

Potatoes

Tabasco® sauce

Tomatillos

Tomatoes

Other

Canned foods (wild salmon in purified water and sardines in olive oil are okay)

Coffee

Processed food

Hydrolyzed yeast (code for MSG)

Canola oil

Rapeseed oil

Safflower oil

Vegetable oil

Sunflower oil

Peanut oil

Partially hydrogenated oils

Milk chocolate

Black tea

Caffeinated teas for the first two months

Chapter 14

Supplements: Discover and Discern What Is Best

In addition to the food you eat there are a number of supplements and lifestyle factors that can assist in functional ketogenic gut repair and support a healthy gut microbiome afterwards. These provide the foundation for a healthy immune system and overall optimal health. The first is proper supplementation.

Frankly, I'm a supplement snob, in that I will only ingest and suggest what I believe to be the highest-quality, cleanest, most effective supplements on the market today. I get results with my patients because I don't waste their time or money on supplements that aren't potent, or that contain toxic excipients.

I don't recommend taking vitamins, because 98 percent of them are synthetic and your body can't (and won't) use them. This may surprise you, but stop and think. There are thousands of phytonutrients, or plant-based nutrients, in vegetables and fruits. When you take a vitamin supplement, it usually contains the 13 basic ones—and most of the time they've been created in a lab. This means your body won't absorb them well, or at all, and you'll likely just pee them out. (This is why your pee is often bright yellow after taking supplements.) Result: expensive urine!

Imagine you have an organic Fuji apple in your hand right now. Look at its beautiful red and green coloring and texture. This apple has about 9,000 phytonutrients in it, all of which work synergistically to benefit the human body. When scientists isolate a single nutrient—say, vitamin C—synthesize it in a lab, and administer a mega-dose, the human body can't assimilate it well because the vitamin is missing the many thousands of other co-nutrients that allow it to be properly absorbed and used. Which means a small amount of natural vitamin C in a plant with all of its other nutrient helpers is more potent than a high-milligram synthetic vitamin pill. Mother Nature really does know what she's doing.

Do *not* purchase probiotics, omega-fatty acids, vitamins, herbs, or any other supplements or natural remedies from a corner market where you pick up your prescriptions, a bargain warehouse, or a large chain store. These stores offer many quality products, but nutritional supplements are categorically not among them. It's important to find a healthcare provider who uses viable and potent professional products and knows what's best for your particular health picture.

Prebiotics and Probiotics

Prebiotics and probiotics are both essential for intestinal microbiota balance, immune function, healthy weight, neurotransmitters, and optimal health. Probiotics are live microorganisms that, when given in small amounts, support you, the host, by improving digestive health, brain chemistry, hormone balance, and immune function. The International Scientific Association for Probiotics and Prebiotics (ISAPP) follows the growing body of scientific studies that demonstrate ways probiotics can benefit human health. These benefits include "reducing antibiotic-associated diarrhea, helping manage digestive symptoms, improving your ability to fight off colds, promoting healthy vaginal and urinary tracts, and improving digestion of lactose. Other benefits include treating infectious diarrhea, and in infants, reducing the risk of eczema, symptoms of colic and necrotizing enterocolitis. Promising targets in initial stages of research include glycemic and weight control and brain function."[88] "Another study notes that specific bacteria or microbial products can help stimulate immune responses."[89]

More simply put, probiotics can help balance immune function.

The particular combination of strains in a probiotic supplement, their viability, and their potency measured in colony-forming units or CFUs, are very important. Probiotic potency commonly ranges from 1 billion to 100 billion CFUs. A diversity of good microbes in your gut is important for your health, and particular strains and combinations of strains have been researched to benefit various health challenges. It is important to cycle different probiotic strains to ensure a healthy diversity of gut flora. There are a few good brands and many awful brands, so please work with a holistic healthcare provider who knows their stuff. I prefer high-potency probiotics of 100 billion CFU per serving. Most need refrigeration, but some are shelf stable.

Some probiotics are best taken with food, and others without. Read the label, and consult a trained holistic healthcare expert in their use. Buyer beware of purchasing from online distributors different from the actual producing company, as they will not guarantee potency and may not ship the product properly with an ice pack. It's best to always purchase a professional probiotic product that has been designed to contain viable, non-competing strains that are acid- and heat-resistant. Most yogurt culture probiotics are destroyed by the acid in your stomach.

Probiotics are also safe for children—though at a lower potency and only those particular strains appropriate for children's guts.

Prebiotics

While not as well-known as probiotics, prebiotics are just as important for maintaining gut health. Prebiotics are non-digestible plant fibers, fermented ingredients, and oligosaccharides that help feed the good bacteria such as *Bifidobacteria* and (to a lesser extent) *Lactobacilli* living in your large intestine and colon.

Prebiotics are different from probiotics in many ways. They are not affected by temperature, stomach acid, or time as probiotics commonly are. Certain probiotics must compete with other bacteria in the gut—including other probiotics—but prebiotics have no such competition.

The benefits of prebiotics include:

- Increased "good" bacteria in the gut—most important of all
- Concomitant decrease in the "bad" unwanted bacteria in the gut
- Increased calcium and magnesium absorption
- Stronger bones, increased bone density
- Strengthened immune system
- Reduced blood triglyceride levels
- Better-controlled weight and appetite due to healthy gut hormonal changes
- Reduced abnormal bacterial leakage through the gut wall ("leaky gut")
- Improved bowel regularity
- Potentially reduced intestinal infections
- Potentially reduced inflammation in the colon walls
- Reduced or cessation of smelly flatus

Prebiotic plant fibers are found in apple skins, artichokes, chicory root, Jerusalem artichokes/sunchokes, leeks, beans, wheat (contains gluten, so avoid), banana (super-high sugar impact, so beware if you have blood sugar imbalances, insulin resistance tendencies, or candida), soy

Please note: The essential amino acids you need for almost every biological process in your body are dependent on your digestive system. Amino acids must be broken down during the digestive process, and identifying and resolving gut issues is imperative for the proper breakdown, absorption, and utilization of the essential amino acids. Trypsin and chymotripsin are two primary pancreatic enzymes used in the breakdown of protein. Gastric pepsin is initially needed for protein digestion, as about 20 percent of protein is broken down in the stomach; the rest is digested in the duodenum and the jejunum of the small intestine. A healthy gut is imperative.

THE SCIENCE
Liposomal Delivery

Many supplements just don't get into your body well, especially if you have any digestive impairment. One solution is to purchase supplements that enter your cells via liposomal delivery. There aren't as many liposomal supplements as we need, but they are coming, and I highly recommend using supplements in this form. Liposomes are made from phospholipids, which are the building blocks of every cell membrane in your body. They encase a nutrient compound, bypassing the normal digestive process, in order to enhance absorption. They can deliver their compound directly into the cell, and have the ability to cross the blood–brain barrier. They further cellular excretion of toxins and also feed the cell membrane, ensuring proper function. Some lyposomals are so easy to absorb, they are the next best thing to an IV.

Buyer beware: Many companies use cheap liposomes, often raw lecithin, that are too large of a molecule and therefore unable to enter the cell. Become an informed consumer, and do your homework on the best products available.

Digestive Enzymes

Digestive enzymes can be critical support tools when beginning comprehensive gut repair. Raw foods contain many important nutrients, but eating raw food all the time can cause digestive trouble. If you already have digestive challenges, you may not be able to tolerate raw food, much less digest and absorb it. And some foods and herbs require cooking to release therapeutic properties.

In TCM, someone with digestive challenges usually does better with an 80 percent cooked/20 percent raw diet. This can eventually shift to 50 percent cooked/50 percent raw depending on the season and your constitution.

Overcooking or microwaving can destroy food enzymes and vital nutrients, rendering your food nutritionally dead, denatured, and lifeless. Taking enzymes increases the nutritive value of your food because they allow you to better break down and absorb nutrients from the food you eat. When there is pancreatic insufficiency, inadequate chewing of food, history of poor nutrition, hidden food sensitivities, poor health, stress, aging, and genetic factors, it's important to support digestion by taking enzymes and help the absorption of nutrients.

CAUTION: If you've had your gallbladder removed

If your gallbladder is gone, you require extra support in order to process the healthy fat you need for a balanced therapeutic ketogenic gut repair plan. You will need digestive enzymes, betaine HCl with pepsin, bile salts (often another name for ox bile, check bile salt source) as directed, and ox bile taken with fatty meals. Make sure to get professional support. Ox bile can give you diarrhea, so start with a low dose like 50–125 mg per dose. If you get diarrhea cut back, reintroduce more slowly, and please consult your doctor. Bile salts can be helpful if you have gallbladder issues or gallstones. Consider reading my Holistic Health Guide on Gallbladder on my website.

There are many digestive enzyme products on the market today, so please consult with a holistic healthcare provider to find one that is right for you.

Betaine Hydrochloride (Betaine HCl)

Almost every person I see has functional lab evidence of hypochlorhydria—low hydrochloric acid (HCl) or stomach acid. Usually, as your gut heals, these markers move into healthy range and tell me your body is making more HCl. Some people can successfully begin producing more HCl on their own, and others must remain on it for longer durations.

Some people must supplement HCl for the rest of their lives, but don't panic. I'm one of those people (due to thyroid issues), and I've found inexpensive and convenient ways to get what I need even when I'm traveling. For example, I keep a small container in my purse with extra enzymes and HCl, so when I'm on the plane and enjoying my delicious home-cooked food (which I also carry), I'm able to digest and absorb it. My fellow passengers often comment about how envious they are that I have such yummy food with me.

HCl makes up about 5 percent of the gastric juices (also known as gastric acid), which is mostly comprised of potassium chloride, or KCl, and sodium chloride, or NaCl. HCl stomach acid and the other gastric juices are essential to help break down your food, which is critical for the absorption of many nutrients, such as protein, iron, zinc, copper, and calcium. Gastric acid itself averages a pH of 1.5 to 3.5, and the mucous membrane of the stomach protects you from that strong acid.

HCl prevents gut microbes from migrating up and colonizing the stomach, and must be present so that you can release and activate the proper enzymes and better digest and absorb your nutrients. Without this, your food is most likely putrefying in your gut, feeding bad bacteria, and causing bloating, gas, and weight gain. HCl also plays the important role of supporting your immune function through its corrosive acid barrier, which kills disease-causing particles and food-borne pathogens (bacteria, viruses, parasites, and so on). For example, people with *Helicobacter pylori* (*H. pylori*) infections have chronic low HCl-levels.

There are three main symptoms of low stomach acid you can look for:

Burping, farting, feeling bloated after meals. Let's get more specific: Do you have several burps shortly after finishing a meal, or burps later that taste and smell bad? Do you experience gas 1–2 hours after eating? Do you get bloated after eating—bloating that lasts for a few hours? Do you have a heavy feeling in your stomach or bloating, like your food just sits there fermenting?

You don't feel good after you eat meat. This is a classic scenario for many people, more women than men. You feel like you're in tune with your body, and you've convinced yourself that meat isn't good for you; however, the likely physiological reason is that *you simply can't digest it*. Your body and mind may reject things they can't properly deal with, but that doesn't mean those things (including meat) aren't necessary building blocks for your tissues and necessary to sustain your health. I gently challenge you to get tested for HCl-sufficiency, if this sounds like you. Or do the self-test explained below.

You experience frequent acid reflux after eating. People take Tums or antacids to reduce stomach acid because they experience acid reflux. But this is the exact *opposite* of what they should be doing. Most people with gastro-esophageal reflux disease (GERD), heartburn, or acid reflux actually have low HCl. Low levels of essential HCl stomach acid lead to conditions that increase intra-abdominal pressure (IAP). When IAP increases, it pushes against the lower esophageal sphincter (LES), which forces the sphincter to open even just a tiny bit. This opening allows for small amounts of stomach acid to touch the esophagus, producing terrible burning and pain. This is mistaken for acid reflux and misprescribed antacids do nothing to cure it.

HCl-supplementation, along with digestive enzymes, a clean diet and lifestyle, and functional gut repair can turn on your body's ability to increase secretion of HCl. Also remember that chewing well is necessary in order to stimulate proper secretion of HCl by the stomach lining.

Betaine HCl Dosing

This is a very individual process. There are many different brands on the market, but I prefer one with added pepsin and/or gentian bitters. I recommend you do the HCl-test to determine your dose.

Caution: NSAIDs and corticosteroids increase the chances of ulcers in the stomach and together with Betaine HCl increase the risk of gastritis. Consult a physician before trying this test or supplementing.

Dosage: Begin by taking one HCl-with-pepsin capsule, approximately 550–650 mg, in the middle of your meal. If you don't notice anything, then you most likely have low HCl. Increase by one capsule per meal, taken in the middle of each meal, until you feel a burning sensation like acid reflux.

For example, you might start with one capsule in the middle of breakfast. For lunch, increase to two capsules in the middle of the meal. For dinner, increase to three capsules in the middle of the meal. For breakfast the next day, increase to four caps in the middle of the meal. For lunch the next day, increase to five capsules in the middle of the meal. For dinner the next day, increase to six capsules in the middle of the meal. For the following breakfast increase to seven capsules, and so on, until you feel a burn.

Once you feel a burn, then decrease your dose by one capsule, and stay on this dose for at least three months. Please work with a holistic healthcare provider to individualize and gain support during this process.

I've had several patients have alternative symptoms/signals that a maximum dose has been reached, such as a tightening in the throat or a tense, almost cramp-like sensation in the stomach.

Some people can wean off or wean down from the HCl, but I always look at follow-up lab findings to see if hypochlorhydria signs disappear or reappear. Wean down over a 10 day period and see how you feel. If symptoms return then add HCl back in. There may be heavy meals or stressful life situations necessitating the continued use of HCl. These factors need to be evaluated by a healthcare provider who is versed in this and can individualize it for you.

Some natural supplements that can help with digestion are apple cider vinegar and digestive bitters. Some people will do well with digestive bitters, and others will need to take an actual supplement of Betaine HCl to help rebalance the pH of the stomach, kill unhealthy microbes, and facilitate healthy digestion. It's a process, and healing can take time. But low stomach acid is quite simple and inexpensive to remedy with supplementation.

Vitamin D3

Vitamin D3 is known as the "sunshine vitamin." It isn't technically a vitamin, because your body can produce it on its own with a little help from the sun, but without the sun (and a few other contributing factors), we don't produce enough. Currently, an estimated 85 percent of people in the US are Vitamin D deficient.

I remember when I was 10 years old. I was living in a suburb of Chicago, and the weather was often overcast—an obvious vitamin D3-deficient area. In addition, when it was sunny, my parents cared for my skin by applying sunscreen. This didn't help, either—it actually blocked my body from performing the vital chemical processes to produce vitamin D in my skin. I also had gut problems, because I wasn't adequately breastfed and had food sensitivities and heavy metal exposure, which meant that my ability to convert vitamin D was impaired. When I fell off the jungle gym, it wasn't a big fall, and I shouldn't have broken any bones, but I fractured my right arm. I suspect that low vitamin D levels were to blame.

There are two forms of Vitamin D: ergocalciferol (vitamin D2) and cholecalciferol (vitamin D3). It used to be thought that they were inter-changeable, but that was based on research done more than 70 years ago on infants and rickets (the childhood vitamin D deficiency disease that causes soft bones prone to fractures and deformities). Between the two, science has shown that vitamin D3 is the preferred form for humans.

Vitamin D3 does so much more than protect your bones and teeth. It's essential for healthy immune function and many other dimensions of health. Its metabolic product is a steroid hormone that regulates over 1,000 genes in the human genome. This means it impacts how your genes express themselves and potentially turn the switch for disease on or off (also known as the field of epigenetics).

Vitamin D3 can also help you avoid:

- Type 1 diabetes
- Cardiovascular disease, including heart attack
- High blood pressure, since Vitamin D3 decreases the production of renin, a hormone believed to play a role in hypertension
- Cancers of the colon, prostate, ovaries, esophagus, and lymphatic system
- Muscle and bone pain
- Broken bones
- Osteoporosis and low calcium absorption
- Autoimmune diseases, such as Hashimoto's thyroiditis, multiple sclerosis, and rheumatoid arthritis
- Allergies—Vitamin D3 helps regulate your immune system.

If you spend 25–35 minutes a day (darker skin needs longer) in the sun, naked, without sunscreen or lotions and without bathing afterward for 24–48 hours, then your D3 levels may rise to functional ranges. If you don't have that much sun exposure, or if you have any gut, skin, liver, kidney, or autoimmune problems, then you need to have your vitamin D3, 25-hydroxy level and 1,25 dihydroxyvitamin D (calcitriol) checked. Vitamin D3, 25-hydroxy is not the active form of Vitamin D3. It's often the only marker checked for D3 status, but adding calcitriol is more comprehensive because this is the usable form of Vitamin D3 in your body.

THE SCIENCE
How Sunshine Works for Your Health

This is how your body converts useble vitamin D3 from sun exposure on your skin:

- Ultraviolet B rays from the sun convert a precursor in your skin (7-dehydrocholesterol) into vitamin D3.
- In the liver, D3 mixes with oxygen and hydrogen to change it into 25-hydroxyvitamin D. This is what most doctors test for in your blood, but it is still the inactive form of vitamin D. I like to test both, when possible.

- The third and final step occurs in the kidneys, where more oxygen and hydrogen molecules attach to 25-hydroxyvitamin D and convert it into its active form, known as 1,25 dihydroxyvitamin D, or calcitriol.

Vitamin D3 levels that are too low *or* too high are unhealthy. Many functional doctors suggest keeping vitamin D3 levels between 50 and 70 ng/ml. The standard acceptable level in Western medicine is between 30 and 100 ng/ml, but 30 ng/ml is too low and 100 is too high. Sun exposure is helpful but often simply not enough. If people are below 45 ng/ml, then I recommend 2,000–10,000 IU per day—proper dosing depends on age, health, and lifestyle factors; lab markers; and latitude—taken with food for two months. If 1,25 dihydroxyvitamin D is high, it can be used as a marker of inflammation.

After that, retest and adjust the dose accordingly.

I have found that 2,000–5,000 IU per day is a solid maintenance dose for most people. Vitamin D3 supplements should be free of excipients and unhealthy oils, such as soy, safflower, and canola. Medium chain triglycerides (MCTs) and olive oil are safe and healthy carriers for vitamin D3.

To get the most out of taking vitamin D3, you also need to consider important mineral cofactors that support your body to properly utilize the D3. These are magnesium, boron, and zinc. Vitamin D3 is fat soluble, so your body doesn't quickly get rid of it if you take too much. It also requires healthy fat digestion in order to absorb it properly.

High levels of vitamin D3, without the proper balance of minerals and vitamins, can lead to toxicity. Vitamin K2 and vitamin A protect us from the toxic effects of vitamin D3. As always, please work with a holistic healthcare provider for appropriate testing and support.

Omega-3 Essential Fatty Acids

The omega-3 essential fatty acids (EFAs)—eicosapentaenoic acid (EPA) and docosahexaenoic acid (DHA)—have anti-inflammatory properties and are important for immune function. The typical Western diet contains a disproportionate amount of omega-6 fatty acids, such as arachidonic acid, which can be pro-inflammatory. You need a higher ratio of omega-3s to balance and counter the inflammatory properties of the omega-6 acids. This decreases the deleterious effects of inflammation from chronic disease and can reduce the risk of cardiovascular disease, neurodegenerative disorders such as Alzheimer's, inflammatory bowel disease, cancer, and autoimmune diseases such as rheumatoid arthritis, Hashimoto's thyroiditis, multiple sclerosis, and lupus.[90]

The media has touted the benefits of omega-3 EFAs for cardiovascular disease, but we're finding it supports the body in many other ways as well. Inflammation causes cellular stress, and omega-3 EFAs not only reduce this stress but can even help cancer patients by positively impacting the anti-tumor functions of the immune system.[91]

Whenever possible, it's important to find a product made from small fish like sardines, rather than large fish like salmon or cod. The larger the fish, the more heavy metals they accumulate. Purchasing products made from fresh oils is imperative. Many commercial fish oils are rancid and can cause your body more harm than good. One way to check is to bite into a capsule. If it tastes super fishy or smells bad, it may be rancid. If you burp up the oil shortly after taking it, then it may also be rancid.

If you purchase anything off the shelf at a health food store, find out where it came from and how long it's been there. If you order something online, know where it came from. If it sat on the tarmac in Phoenix, Arizona, in the middle of summer, it most likely is bad and no longer therapeutic.

Glutathione

Glutathione is the mother of antioxidants because it fights free radical damage and helps regenerate other antioxidants, such as vitamin C and vitamin E. Glutathione is excellent at helping you detoxify and eliminate heavy metals by supporting your liver, kidneys, and intestines—all important organs of detoxification. It supports immune function, especially the proper functioning of your white blood cells and T cell lymphocytes. It helps decrease oxidative stress and inflammation in the entire body and greatly supports gut repair. It is especially useful in the recovery from oxidative stress-induced diseases and the prevention of disease.

Antioxidants help you decrease the effects of aging, exposure to toxic chemicals, damaging metabolic byproducts, long-distance sports that cause increased oxidative stress and tissue damage, and stress. Research has found it aids in detoxification of heavy metals, positively impacts the brain, and aids in tissue repair. Some brands have a sulfur smell and taste, which they claim is normal but can be an indication of a poor product. Some glutathione supplements contain phospholipids derived from soy, but there is no soy protein, and the science shows it does not trigger immune reactions in soy-sensitive individuals, nor is it goitrogenic or estrogenic, so it's safe.

Glutathione is difficult to absorb and assimilate, so choose a liposomal liquid delivery or an IV push. Not all liposomals are created equally. Many have liposomes that are too large and can't actually penetrate the cell wall to deliver the nutrient. It's important to work with a trained healthcare provider who knows their stuff. An IV push can be done by a skilled naturopath, versed in these kinds of methods. I highly recommend IV pushes in the beginning of gut repair to get quick antioxidant support that will bypass any digestive challenges in absorption or commit to taking a liposomal glutathione.

Colostrum

Colostrum is the yellowish pre-breast milk fluid secreted by females right before and after birth in mammals. You may be thinking that I advise avoiding dairy—and I do. But this is different. Colostrum is known for modulating (regulating, balancing) the immune response. Immune-modulating factors help maintain healthy immune function while mediating autoimmune dysfunction. Colostrum contains antibodies or immunoglobulins that offer protection from invading pathogens, bacteria, viruses, toxins, and fungi. It has enhanced bioavailability (ease of absorption) and supports assimilation of nutrients in the digestive tract.

Colostrum has biologically active, anti-aging growth factors that help stimulate cellular and tissue growth, might reverse damage from disease and aging, stimulate protein synthesis, and can affect neurotransmitters to improve moods and mental acuity.

In his book *Colostrum: Life's First Food*, Daniel Clark writes that bovine colostrum "rebuilds the immune system, destroys viruses, bacteria, and fungi, and accelerates healing of all body tissue, while helping with weight loss and builds lean muscle, while slowing down and reversing aging." A 2007 study by a group of researchers in San Valentino found that "colostrum, both in healthy subjects and high-risk cardiovascular patients, is at least three times more effective than vaccination to prevent flu and is very cost-effective."[92] Working with a company that ethically collects colostrum is essential. There are only a few companies that collect only after the calves have had their fill but within six hours of birth, so it's fresh. It is ideal to begin with small doses of ¼ teaspoon twice a day. It should be taken without food, between meals. You can gradually increase dose to a full teaspoon or two, 2–3 times a day. It's a powder, so let it dissolve in your mouth. Don't breathe in, or you can choke on the powder. It will stick to your teeth, so have a little water afterwards.

Cannabinoids

Recent research is celebrating the anti-inflammatory properties of medicinal-grade cannabis. It has been proven to decrease inflammation in neuroinflammatory diseases and autoimmune diseases.

Autoimmune liver disease and viral hepatitis are serious health problems worldwide. According to Hedge et al., "natural cannabinoids such as Δ9-tetrahydrocannabinol (THC) effectively modulate immune cell function, and they have shown therapeutic potential in treating inflammatory diseases."[93] Cannabinoids have also been shown to directly suppress autoimmune-related inflammation of the central nervous system,[94] while inducing apoptosis or cell death of certain cancer cells.[95] This potent herb has significant health benefits!

THE SCIENCE
CANNABIS AND INFLAMMATION

According to a 2015 article in the *Journal of Neuroimmune Pharmacology*, cannabinoids, the cannabis constituents, are known to possess anti-inflammatory properties, but the mechanisms involved are not understood. In one study it was shown that the main psychoactive cannabinoid, Δ-9-tetrahydrocannabinol (THC), and the main nonpsychoactive cannabinoid, cannabidiol (CBD), markedly reduce the Th17 phenotype, which is known to be increased in inflammatory autoimmune pathologies such as multiple sclerosis.[96]

Cannabinoids have been found to have both neuroprotectant and antioxidant properties, which makes them a strong candidate in the treatment of oxidative stress-related diseases. These include autoimmune disorders, inflammation, work-out recovery for endurance athletes, most chronic and degenerative disease patterns, and anti-aging support. Their neuroprotectants are useful in treating neurodegenerative diseases like dementia, Type 3 diabetes (dementia brought about by high blood sugar, causing shrinking of the white matter of the brain), and Alzheimer's and Parkinson's diseases. There are various forms of cannabinoids. Cannabidiol, for example, is nonpsychoactive, and therefore avoids the potential toxicity that occurs with psychoactive cannabinioids at high doses.

In layman's terms we can say cannabinoids are great antioxidants and anti-inflammatories, and they can help balance immune function and protect your brain. You can obtain THC-free, pure medicinal cannabinoid tinctures online (CBD). THC is the psychoactive and illegal (in some places) part of cannabis. Cannabinoids are now on many grocery store shelves next to vitamin D3 and omega-3 fish oils for their immune-modulating, antioxidant, and anti-inflammatory properties.

Additional Supplements for Gut Health

I've included the following gut supporting supplements because of their therapeutic value. However, remember that you are unique; what works for your best friend may not work for you. You can try various combinations of these herbs if you are not taking any prescription drugs. Be careful of drug/herb interactions, and please consult a holistic healthcare provider to find what works best for you. Generally speaking, all these are considered "safe."

L-glutamine

L-glutamine is an amino acid that has been proven to build lean muscle and heal leaky gut. B12 helps control glutamine build-up in the body, so if you're taking L-glutamine long-term, it's wise to also take methylcobalamin or hydroxolcobalamin, the most bioavailable forms of B12, in the form of a quick painless injection once a month or by using cutaneous patches. The injection must be into a muscle, so find a doctor who uses the proper size needle. I inject myself in my thigh muscle using a 1-inch needle (1 inch equals 2.54 cm). Liposomal B12 or sublingual tablets of B12 are also acceptable, but you won't absorb very much from the tablets.

As long as your nutritional and lifestyle plan avoids gut-damaging things, L-glutamine acts like "multi-purpose filler" for your gut, helping to seal the tight-junction gaps and eventually eliminate leaky gut. Research shows that it improves your energy while increasing your athleticism. It aids detoxification by cleansing the body of high levels of ammonia, and helps to heal ulcerative colitis.[97] A hospital study found that it reduces intestinal permeability.[98] It also helps the body regulate IgA immune response, often found in food sensitivities.

Dosage is 1–18 grams per day mixed with a few ounces of water or aloe vera juice. Drink on an empty stomach. It is great to take after a workout.

Marshmallow Root

Marshmallow root is mucilaginous and quite soothing to the digestive tract. It decreases inflammation and lubricates the intestines. It's best taken as a cold infusion. Begin with the dried root, add it to a glass jar of water, cover, and place in your refrigerator overnight. I usually use a large, 32-ounce/1-liter canning jar and about one-third to one-half of a cup of dried herb. By the next morning, you will have your cold infusion of marsh-mallow root. It will remain good in the refrigerator for about 10 days. When you've consumed half of it, you can add water to top up. It will be slightly diluted, but still plenty therapeutic.

Dosage: Begin with 2–4 ounces or 60–120 ml twice a day, preferably on an empty stomach.

Aloe Vera

Aloe vera is a popular plant for skin conditions, including sunburn, but research points to its digestive health benefits as well. The *British Journal of General Practice* notes its soothing effects for symptoms of ulcers of the stomach and intestines, irritable bowel syndrome, colitis, and other digestive inflammatory problems. It helps soothe and decrease inflammation in the gastrointestinal system and can help lubricate the intestines.[99]

Because aloe vera helps heal the digestive tract, it makes sense that it also positively impacts the immune system. Aloe vera possesses antifungal, antiviral, and antibacterial properties that support the immune system to combat pathogens more easily and to detoxify the body.[100] It can also help reduce the symptoms of seasonal allergies, rheumatoid arthritis, and constipation.

Caution: Be careful if you're taking blood sugar-lowering medication, as aloe vera may increase the actions of that medication. It may cause potassium loss if you're taking diuretics and can also cause diarrhea.

Tulsi

Tulsi, or holy basil, is one of the most sacred plants of India. It's in the mint family and closely related to the basil plant. Tulsi naturally relieves stress and anxiety while acting as a potent antioxidant, antibacterial, antifungal and anti-inflammatory. It's soothing to the digestive system and has even been used to treat ulcers.[101, 102]

Tulsi has traditionally been used for the common cold, bronchitis, and fevers. I love caffeine-free tulsi teas—tulsi tea bags are convenient for travel and guests. You can add therapeutic herbs and spices, such as mint, rose, cinnamon, and licorice (but don't use licorice if you have high blood pressure).

Peppermint

Peppermint is soothing to the digestive tract and is commonly used for conditions like irritable bowel syndrome (IBS). It can be taken as a tea or enteric-coated capsules or tablets, which allows it to pass through the stomach to the upper regions of the GI tract where it soothes. Peppermint acts as a smooth muscle relaxant in the lower GI. Its aroma and flavor are soothing to the nervous system, which you now know is directly connected to your GI tract. You may even consider a drop or two of pure organic peppermint essential oil added to your water bottle. It doubles as a great breath freshener.

Peppermint is well tolerated by most people, but too many capsules can have adverse effects. Please consult with a holistic healthcare provider for dosage support.

Chamomile

Chamomile has been used in newborns to soothe colic. It's a common herb and is known as the "mother of the gut." It is antimicrobial and anti-inflammatory, and possesses antispasmodic properties that make it useful for acute and chronic distress. It's been found to calm the central nervous system due to a chemical compound in the flowers called apigenin, which is linked to GABA receptors in the brain.

Fennel

Preparations of fennel leaves and seeds have also been used to treat digestive symptoms and even help colicky infants. It helps and prevents heartburn, constipation, gas, and bloating. You can make a tea from it and use the bulbs in stir-fries and salads. Some sources have found fennel to stimulate digestive enzyme secretion. Chewing on the dried seeds can support digestion and freshen your breath after a meal.

Ginger

Ginger root has a long history as a digestive aid. It's been used in TCM for warming the spleen and aiding in the resolution of dampness for thousands of years. Ginger reduces nausea, vomiting, motion sickness, and morning sickness in pregnancy, and calms the digestive tract. It has anti-inflammatory properties as well for the joints, but it must be used for about eight weeks before the effects are noticed. Ginger root is meant to be steeped, not fully boiled. If you purchase organic, then you need not peel off the skin.

Dosage: I like chopping the root—about 2 inches' or 5 cm worth—into quarter-inch chunks, adding them to a pot containing 4 cups (1 l) of water, then heating to just below a simmer for about 45 minutes and letting cool on the stove. Sip the tea throughout the day, and store in the refrigerator for use the following day.

Digestive Bitters

Digestive bitters, or Swedish bitters, are a combination of herbs that support the secretion of digestive enzymes and soothe, decrease inflammation, and support the epithelial lining of the GI tract. Elixirs of bitter herbs have been used in Europe throughout history and touted as a "cure-all." Bitters can reduce bloating and gas by helping move things through the digestive process more thoroughly. Bitters also curb sugar cravings, support your liver, balance your appetite, relieve constipation, and alleviate nausea. Depending on the combination of herbs, bitters are safe, and they are often used for morning sickness.

Vitamins

I don't usually recommend vitamins because almost all of them are synthetic, which means they are less bioavailable. There are very few vine-ripened, organic vegetable and fruit powders that meet my high standards. Even organic foods are often picked early and not allowed to ripen on the vine; about 50 percent of the nutrients enter the vegetable or fruit in the last 20 percent of the growing period. Therefore, most organic produce found in stores is missing about 50 percent of its vital nutrients. This holds true for food-based supplements as well.

I prefer whole food vitamins; some are even fermented. This can be beneficial for absorption unless you have high histamine responses. I prefer fruit powders to be sugar-free, which means the sugar is extracted, making it safe for people with cancer, diabetes, and candida. There is only one company that I've found that has the gold standard of research on their product. This means double-blind, peer-reviewed, placebo-controlled, independent, and published in peer-reviewed journals. Look for studies done on the actual product rather than a general study about Vitamin C or antioxidants. It is legal to take random research and plug it onto any product and use it to promote the efficacy of that product, although this doesn't seem ethical to me. If you are doing gut repair, consider getting a series of IV nutrient infusions, such as Myer's Cocktails, or begin taking a well-researched liposomal vitamin complex.

Chapter 15

The Importance of Hydration, Sleep, and Exercise

Our bodies are made up of 75–85 percent water at any given time. We require water to sustain life for basic metabolic functioning, to energize the body, to maintain health, detoxify, and heal. Without water, many systems of the body are compromised and begin to break down, often without notice, until tissue damage has accumulated sufficiently to grab one's full attention.

The Importance of Hydration

A cornerstone of any gut-repair program is hydration. Dehydration is a primary cause of ill health. You must drink plenty of pure water! Tea and coffee are not water and don't count. Neither do soda water, tonic water, and various flavored waters from the store.

As a baseline, you need to drink one-thirtieth of your body weight in pure spring water every day. That's the minimum amount for a contented couch potato. If you're active—if you work, exercise, have stress, or drink herbal or green tea or caffeinated beverages—you need more. An easy way to calculate the amount of water you need is to divide your body weight in pounds by two and add 16 ounces more to that number; that gives you the necessary number of ounces of water you need every day. For example, if you weigh 150 pounds, you need 75 ounces of water daily. The metric calculation: divide your weight in kg by 30, then add 0.5, and that is the number of liters you need daily. If you exercise, take medications, drink tea or coffee, or have stress, add *at least* another 8–16 ounces or 250–500 ml.

Dehydrators

Caffeine, coffee and tea, sports drinks, sugar, alcohol, medications, an arid environment, electrolyte imbalances, stress, and physical activity dehydrate the body. To compensate, drink the right amount of water between meals on an empty stomach. Consider starting the day off right with half to 1 quart of water upon rising (8–16 ounces/250–500 ml), at least 30 minutes before breakfast. This can promote a bowel movement and begin hydrating you immediately. Drink more water between meals. I caution you not to drink too much water at meals, only a small glass for supplements, because it dilutes stomach acid and inhibits digestion.

Many forms of inflammation can be traced back to chronic dehydration. Chronic pain can be a sign of dehydration. Arthritis, which means "joint inflammation," can be worsened by dehydration because cartilage consists largely of water. When it begins to dry out, it can't glide as well and becomes damaged, leading to pain. Histamine responses to the environment or food allergens are also strong indicators of dehydration. Primary (idiopathic) hypertension has no known cause but can be the result of chronic dehydration. As dehydration sets in, blood pressure rises to keep vital cells hydrated. Consider reading *Your Body's Many Cries for Water: You're Not Sick; You're Thirsty: Don't Treat Thirst with Medications* by Dr. F. Batmanghelidj.[103]

The Right Water Matters

It's also important to drink the right kind of water. Tap water has a long list of disadvantages, including contamination from prescription drug residues and heavy metals. Toxic chemicals are often used to disinfect the water, and contaminants like copper, bromine and chlorine, toxic residues of pesticides, herbicides, plastics, and fluoride are the norm.

Distilled water can leach vital minerals out of your body, a process known as chelation. It may be useful during a short cleanse but not long term. There are also problems with reverse osmosis (RO), which is by far the most common filtering method. RO removes most chemicals and minerals but doesn't seem to hydrate the body well. (In my work with people who drink a lot of RO water, their labs still show signs of dehydration.) In addition, pre and post filters can quickly become contaminated with viruses and bacteria. Short-term use during travel is acceptable, and RO systems will render contaminant-free water.

The best way to filter water is with a slow-working carbon filter. Remember, filters must be changed often, and the vast majority of carbon filters are not designed to remove fluoride, nitrates, sodium, inorganics such as lead and mercury, or microbiological contaminants like coliform and cysts like Giardia and Cryptosporidium. However, high-density, solid carbon .5 micron block filters (such as ones used by Multipure) handle a great deal more than the cheaper models. Be sure to read the labels and find out what the particular filter is designed to remove.

The best water is wild, which means it comes from a fresh spring. If you don't have a spring nearby, then purchase real spring water, preferably bottled in glass.

It's important not only to drink clean water but also to bathe with it. You might consider installing a whole-house water filtration system or specialized shower filter. It's a solid investment toward better health. Finally, avoid the fancy bottled waters—most of it is glorified tap water at best. Don't be fooled by labels touting its "alkalinizing" properties.

Finally, try to drink from glass or stainless steel containers whenever possible.

The Importance of Sleep

The way you sleep affects how you feel during waking hours. Quantity and quality matter! Loss of sleep can slowly impact your health over time, or it can hit you in an instant.

Ongoing sleep deprivation has been linked to high blood pressure, cardiovascular disease, stroke, and diabetes. Sleep helps your brain work properly and therefore improves learning, attention, and creativity.[104] Chronic lack of sleep can slow metabolism, alter hormones that regulate appetite, and make you gain weight. As some of you have already experienced, sleep loss can cause irritability and mood swings. Sleep deprivation decreases immune function and can even contribute to certain kinds of cancers.

You also need adequate *quality* sleep every night. For most adults, 8–10 hours of sleep is about right. Children need more: 11–12 hours per night; while teenagers require 9–11 hours of good sleep every night. Limited or poor-quality sleep can impact your health without your initial awareness. Unless they're chronic insomniacs, most people don't even recognize they have sleep deficiencies.

What time of night you fall asleep is also important. Working a swing shift or a graveyard shift negatively affects your body's circadian rhythms, possibly leading to cognitive impairment over time.[105] If you're on such a schedule, do your best to have it changed or get support to stay balanced.

It's best to get to sleep no later than 10 p.m., except for teenagers, whose internal clocks are actually different during their developmental years. They tend to stay up later and need to sleep in longer. Unfortunately, schools have not yet embraced the science behind this phenomenon.

Create healthy sleep attitudes (aka "sleep hygiene") by taking time to slow down in the evenings. Relaxing and down-regulating your nervous system is important. Find whatever helps you to de-stress, and practice it. Meditation, prayer, deep breathing, music, yoga, art, reading, sipping herbal tea, a walk out in nature, cuddling with a loved one, giving and receiving massages and foot rubs, playing with a pet, and journaling are a few ideas to get you started. Avoid overly stimulating activities, such as gossiping on the phone or internet, video games, intense exercise, or watching violent movies or television shows, including the news.

If you're a party-goer, consider staying home more often and away from loud bars, concerts, and heated political debates. There are certainly times to let your hair down and have fun, but plan accordingly, so that your needs for relaxation, rest, and rejuvenation are met first. People who tend to chronically overdo it are more likely to have digestive and immune dysfunction.

The Importance of Exercise

Exercise is an important component of any comprehensive health and well-being plan. Cardiovascular training, resistance or weight training, and some kind of stretching, Pilates, Gyrotonic, and yoga practice will address most of the body's fitness needs.

The benefits of exercise have been scientifically proven again and again. It reduces body fat, increases muscle mass, strengthens the cardiovascular system, increases HDL cholesterol (the good one), decreases your risk of diabetes and Alzheimer's, lowers blood sugar, increases energy and lung function, and releases stress and tension in the body and mind. If you stick with it, your aerobic capacity will increase, along with oxygenation of your blood and brain, leading to more alertness. Increasing your aerobic capacity will also make you feel younger. You'll experience the benefit of increased endorphins, which are released by the central nervous system and pituitary gland during exercise and sexual activity. These are the "feel good" chemicals that actually mimic morphine—the chemicals responsible for the "runner's high" you often hear about.

Start easy. Begin by taking a 15-minute daily walk. Studies show even 15 minutes can elevate mood, stimulate metabolism, and increase circulation and oxygenation of your cells, muscles, and brain. Gradually increase the duration to 30 minutes and incorporate a few easy hills. You might want to walk with a friend or family member or listen to an audio book to help with motivation and accountability.

New research shows that doing short bursts of intense effort yields more benefit with less oxidative stress than longer workouts of varying intensity. Interval training might begin, for example, with a five-minute warm-up with a medicine ball or stationary bike. Next comes 30 seconds of intense exercise, followed by 30 seconds of lighter recovery activity. For example, run, cycle, or swim as fast and as hard as you can for 30 seconds, then jog, spin, or swim at a slower, more moderate pace. During the interval go fast and hard. Push yourself. (You shouldn't be able to speak during the interval because you're breathing too hard!)

You can do stationary bike, jumping jacks, run with high knees and arms extended out from your sides, burpees, jump rope, or jump up and hit your knees in mid-air. If you're just beginning, do only three sets of this and then a five-minute cool-down. Do this three or four times a week. After a week or two, consider increasing the interval to 40 seconds of intense exercise followed by 40 seconds of a slower pace. Do five sets. After another week or two, increase to 60 seconds of intense exercise, followed by a 60-second moderate- to low-intensity exercise, and do five to 10 sets, gradually increasing to as many as 15–20 sets over time. This is a very simplified version of high-intensity interval training (HIIT).

Exercise is an act of self-love. It's an important key in both the prevention and treatment of every disease pattern. You have the power to choose health! But please, first check with your primary healthcare provider before embarking on any exercise program.

Chapter 16

Self-Awareness and Introspection Exercises

Increasing self-awareness is an important part of my Functional Ketogenic Gut Repair Program. Honestly, we don't know what we don't know, and there are ways to develop self-awareness, which will speed healing.

Mental, physical, emotional, spiritual, and energetic awareness should be part of your relationship with your body every bit as much as your relationship with other people and your environment. And everyone "senses" differently. Some people are more naturally aware of sensations in their body. Some are more aware of their emotions and thoughts. Other people sense visually, and still others sense best through the medium of hearing.

All of these are important, and I invite you to identify both your strengths and weaknesses when it comes to your own inner awareness. Taking steps to develop your awareness will help shine a light on patterns and beliefs you've learned that no longer serve you, possibly keeping your body stuck in illness.

Food Addiction and Comfort Eating

If you're a comfort eater, you stuff your feelings and soothe your emotions with food and beverages, rewarding yourself with food treats. I get it; my mom was a comfort eater. I understand the kinds of experiences and patterns that trigger comfort eating. Problems with weight, trauma, low self-esteem, and childhood abuse are only a few. And I have seen these patterns getting passed down generation to generation.

The reason I'm telling you all this is because I want you to know that I understand the cycle of pleasure and pain that you may be experiencing as a comfort eater—the pleasure to be had eating the chocolate cake and the pain of the guilt and the symptoms it causes after you eat it, bouncing from the high you feel because your dopamine receptors just got a sugar hit (like taking heroin) to the depression that comes from the self-sabotage.

It takes self-reflection to realize that the sugar and other treats are creating a barrier between you and the things you don't wish to feel or experience—that what you're doing is engaging in a kind of self-protection action, learned early in life, which may or may not truly be serving your adult self.

Various kinds of talk therapy may help you identify the root of the patterns; however, they likely won't help you change the eating pattern itself. Many different healing modalities I've listed in this book can though, and I encourage you to explore and identify what works for you.

Practices

The exercises that follow will help you begin your self-awareness healing journey around food and health. Self-Awareness Practice no. 1 is a step-by-step process for identifying comfort-eating patterns. Self-Awareness Practice no. 2 is a three-step, question-and-answer exercise designed to give you profound insight into your relationship with food, nutrition, and health.

Self-awareness is a rich topic, and I can't possibly touch upon everything I'd like to in this one small section. These two exercises will help you get to know yourself in a different way. Please consider this a little snack, something to whet your appetite for more freedom in your life, peace in your heart, health in your body, and joy in your relationships.

Self-Awareness Practice no. 1

- Begin by setting an intention to remember your wholeness and to connect to your fullest expression of your highest and most beautiful self, then create a statement that reflects this intention. I state mine like this: *I am whole and beautiful, feeling blissful.*
- Now contemplate how it would feel to completely embody your wholeness: feeling connected, beautiful, loving, and joyful. You can use my statement or create your own.
- **Warning:** do not create an intention about something you want to get rid of or something you are trying to push away. Make it a positive statement, not a negative one.
- As best you can, relax into the state of feeling whole, beautiful, and blissful (or whatever qualities spell wholeness and inner beauty to you).

- Next, identify a pattern. The next time you are under stress, notice if your body and mind direct you to food. (If so, I'm guessing it isn't very nutrient dense or healthy food!).
- Observe the physical, mental, and emotional pull to soothe your stress by eating and/or drinking.
- Pause and take five deep breaths that you can feel all the way down into the bottoms of your feet.
- Allow your mind to travel back in time. Ask yourself: *When was the first time I felt this way? When was the first time I soothed myself this way? How old was I? Who was around? What was happening?*
- Shine light on the origins of this pattern without blame or shaming yourself or anyone else. Know that everyone is always doing their very best with the tools they have, and that most of us haven't been given any tools to deal with life at all! Take a moment to write down any insights you may have.
- Take a journey through your life from that first time into the present, and note how this pattern has served you throughout your life. (Trust me, there are gifts in this pattern, even if you haven't seen them yet.) Find the blessings and write these down. Send gratitude to yourself at the age in which the pattern began all the way to the present.
- Next, identify all the various reasons why this pattern no longer serves you, why it perhaps causes you pain and suffering. Write these down and again surround them with gratitude and love.
- Find the pattern or sensation in your body that is associated with this pattern of handling stress (or whatever kind of situation triggers comfort eating). When you feel stress (or have a difficult experience), *where* do you feel the urge to comfort eat? Where is it in your body? What is its size, shape, color, texture? What is the quality of the sensation? Is it hot, cold, big, small, tight, empty, sharp, dull, and so on?
- Go into the sensation. What emotion(s) is hiding beneath the sensation in your body? What beliefs or thoughts are associated with the sensation? Is there a voice and words associated with the sensation? Is it your voice speaking these beliefs to you? Or is it someone else's voice—perhaps a past caregiver or teacher, or someone else?
- Listen to that voice as an observer, not taking this voice seriously, but rather observing it from a place of gratitude that it is finally being heard. Heightening your awareness of this voice and what it has to say will eventually lessen its grasp on you, as long as you don't take it personally. So, observe the voice without judgment or shame.

- Move the energy of the voice/feeling/pattern out of your body in ways that feel good to you. You may shake it out, dance it, yell something, cry. Whatever. There are no rules, and the sky is the limit! Don't be afraid! Allow the all-knowing and divine part of yourself to guide you.
- Pay attention to how the energy wants to move. You may notice that it wants to stay a little longer and develop a connection to your heart or other body part. It may want to speak to another part of you. It may want to leave immediately. It may even give you a visual for how it wants to exit your body—through which body part and in what form. Remain as present as you can. Trust that your body and soul know how to heal.
- Now relax, breathe, and completely release all expectations. Just be here now, breathing and being. You are whole and beautiful, feeling blissful.

Self-Awareness Practice no. 2

It is a fascinating and revealing process to explore your own internal experience of food. It's also a healing journey.

Remember, we don't know what we don't know. I highly recommend that you take the time to explore your connection to food and health through the following three sets of questions. They are specifically designed to give you deep insight into your own patterns and programs around food, health, and nutrition by looking at those things through three different lenses:

- The personal lens "I": your subjective views about food, health, and nutrition
- The subjective lens "you": your group (family/community) subjective views about food, health, and nutrition
- The objective lens "we": how your thoughts and actions around food, nutrition, and health affect the whole (the nation/world).

I suggest getting a pen and paper and writing your answers to all three sets of questions down. That way you can go back over the information and learn from it—even expand on it as new insights arise.

Please note: there are no right or wrong answers—no right or wrong ways to appreciate food, share meals, or sustain your physical body with nutrients. However, broadening your awareness can be insightful and regenerative.

Now, let's explore your answers to the above in more detail.

First-Person Perspective "I"

- What is your personal experience with food, health, and nutrition? What is your direct experience with food, tastes/flavors, and textures? Are you aware of chewing, flavors, textures, and temperatures of the foods you consume? Do you enjoy eating? Do you savor your food? What kind of foods and tastes and textures do you like?
- Do you wolf your food down unthinking? Do you eat while you're distracted by your computer, phone, news programs, music, conversation, magazines, books, or especially the television during meals?
- When did you become aware of your health and the value of nutrition? What were the circumstances that informed this new awareness?
- What were you taught to believe about food, nutrition, and health from others, and what do you value about these teachings? Is food fun, medicinal, a stressor, a place of pain and suffering, numbing medicine, or something to control or be controlled by?
- You've learned various habitual ways of caring for yourself with food. Is food simply sustenance, or do you use it to soothe or suppress emotions like anxiety? How often do you notice yourself doing this food soothing?
- What are the main triggers that elicit food soothing? From where/who do you think you learned this?
- How do you see food serving your highest good?

Second-Person Perspective "You"

Expand your awareness from your individual experience, beliefs, and understandings of food, into the collective perspective, the *cultural* experience of food. Ask yourself the following questions:

- How have your food choices been informed by family, community, and cultural values? What does your family value in regards to food and nutrition?
- What rituals do your family practice with regard to food preparation and mealtimes? Consider these elements: What times of day do you eat meals? What locations inside or outside the home do you use for cooking and eating? How much time do you spend preparing food? Which people participate in food preparation? What peripheral activities (talking, singing, background music, or television) occur during cooking and eating? What special dishes, place settings, or center pieces are present at the table? What particular foods or drinks are always served with meals, and in what order? Where do people sit?

What is the sequence in which people are served? Does the meal begin with a prayer or blessing, and who presides? Are mealtimes treated with reverence, indifference, or irreverence? What happens after the meal? Who cleans up?

- When gathered together, what do you notice about how others experience food? Is their focus on the food? On socializing with others at the table? On socializing with others on mobile devices? On their own thoughts?

- How do your current rituals compare with those when you were growing up? Have you perpetuated or discontinued any particular dining or food choice rituals you learned from your family? Why or why not? Have you invented or adopted new rituals? Do you or your family have a ritual of fasting? Do you or your family have celebration rituals? How does this shape your relationship with food?

- Have you ever eaten food in a foreign country with different customs? What did you notice about their values around food? How do they compare with yours? If you haven't experienced dining in a foreign country, I encourage you to go to an authentic foreign restaurant. Perhaps Ethiopian, Indian, Thai, or Chinese, and notice cultural variations in food and drink selection, table and utensil setup, portion sizes, ambiance, and eye contact. Do any of these attract or repel you? What past experience might have informed your reaction? See if you can spot how other influences (especially from your own culture) might have seeped into the foreign culture.

- How does geography impact cultural values of food? People on the American West Coast eat differently from people who live on the East Coast, or in the Midwest or South. What factors account for these variations? How do these factors influence culture, or in turn, how does culture influence these factors?

Third-Person Perspective "We"

Expand your awareness from individual, family, community, and culture outward to include the systems that support the production, evaluation, and transportation of the food you purchase and consume:

- Consider the impact of your food choices on your body, family, community, and the greater environment—Earth. To what kind of system are you contributing? Where do you grow or purchase food, and how does this impact your community? Do you eat organic, free-range, pastured, genetically modified foods, local foods?

- What informs your food choices? Individual food preferences? Habit? Culture? Affordability? Availability? Climate? Geography?
- How do your food and health choices impact your local community economically?
- What informs your choice of healthcare? Conventional versus alternative? Convenience of access? Knowledge? Experience? Affordability? Insurance coverage? Referral? What systems are you supporting, and how does this impact the future variety, availability, and structure of healthcare choices for yourself and others?

These exercises offer just a little taste of the kind of vast journey you can take when you dive into the arena of self-awareness! I believe it will make you a much more informed consumer, and therefore, an active and empowered participant in your nutritional and health needs.

PART IV

The Food

Chapter 17

Your A–Z Food Guide

This section is dedicated to informing and inspiring you about the therapeutic power of gastronomy and is meant to complement the recipe section that follows. I hope this helps you appreciate how food is truly medicine and to share what you learn with your family and friends.

I've chosen to include Traditional Chinese Medicine (TCM) actions and indications to enhance the Western medical perspective on nutrient content. TCM looks at flavor, temperature, color, and the season in which a food is grown and harvested to determine which *meridians* (energy pathways) and organs it will affect and what imbalances it will harmonize.

I've avoided overwhelming you with information by not including every caloric detail, and have instead chosen to bring specific nutrients in particular foods to your attention in order to best support your Functional Ketogenic Gut Repair Program journey. Make sure you've done comprehensive food sensitivity and reactivity testing, so that you can choose which of the following foods will work best for your body.

Agar

Agar is from Japan, where it's known as *kanten*. Agar is the mucilage of several species of seaweed. In Traditional Chinese Medicine, agar is very cooling in nature, with a slightly sweet flavor. As a result, agar helps reduce inflammation and has a cooling effect on heat conditions, especially those affecting the lungs and heart, such as bronchitis with yellow phlegm. It promotes digestion and is a mild laxative. It also affects the liver and can help carry toxins and even radioactive waste out of the body. Some people have reported that it assists in weight loss.

Apricots

In Traditional Chinese Medicine, apricots are neutral in temperature with a sweet-and-sour flavor. They help produce fluids, and are often used to treat thirst and dryness in the throat and lungs. They are high in fiber, vitamin A, and potassium. They have a relatively short season, from the end of May through June or July, so get them vine ripened when you can.

Arugula

Arugula, or rocket, has bitter and spicy flavors that nourish the heart. Its green color supports the liver and gallbladder.
It's a rich source of certain phytochemicals, such as indoles, thiocyanates, sulforaphane, and isothiocyanates, thus inhibiting the growth of certain types of cancer, such as prostate, breast, cervical, and ovarian. It's a rich source of vitamins A, B, C, and K, beta-carotene, and folates.

Asparagus

In Traditional Chinese Medicine, asparagus is thermally slightly warming and tastes slightly pungent and bitter. It may stimulate urination and helps to alleviate cough, mucus discharge, and various skin eruptions. It also contains inulin, and therefore supports *Bifidobacteria* and *Lactobacilli*

in the large intestine. This can aid in nutrient absorption, decrease the risk of allergies, and lower the risk of colon cancer.

Recent studies show that fresh asparagus contains glutathione, a powerful antioxidant. Asparagus contains vitamins B1, B2, B3, and B6, folate, choline, biotin, and pantothenic acid, necessary for healthy sugar and starch metabolism, thus helping maintain healthy blood sugar levels while lowering homocysteine levels. Homocysteine is a marker of overall health and nutrition—a toxic amino acid that must be kept under control. High levels are an indicator of cardiovascular disease and other disease processes.

Asparagus can be eaten raw or lightly cooked, but it should be consumed within two days of purchase. If needed, wrap the ends in moistened paper towel to preserve freshness. Try it in a salad or with a dip using a recipe from this book. It should be a vibrant green color when cooked, not mushy and light brown. Nutrients are destroyed by overcooking.

Avocados

In Traditional Chinese Medicine, avocados are cooling in thermal nature, sweet in flavor, and build yin, or blood. The avocado is a fruit, not a vegetable (fruits have seeds or pits, but veggies do not), and they are full of wonderful enzymes and rich in healthy fats. They contain copper, which helps form red blood cells, and they help harmonize the liver and lubricate the intestines. Avocados provide nearly 20 essential nutrients, including vitamin K, potassium, B vitamins, folate, lecithin, lutein (an important antioxidant), and fat-soluble vitamin E, an antioxidant that protects the body tissue from damage caused by free radicals. (Free radicals harm cells, tissues, and organs, thus aging us more rapidly and causing degenerative disease.)

Avocados contain a very digestible protein, and they have more than 80 percent good monounsaturated fat, which can help lower LDL (bad) cholesterol and boost HDL (good) cholesterol levels (like an intense interval workout!). Avocados are naturally anti-inflammatory and provide an excellent fat for the brain, muscles, skin, hair, and nails, while supporting sustained energy production. They can also help balance blood sugar, and are thus a superfood to include when changing over to a ketogenic rather than a glucose-based diet.

Basil

In Traditional Chinese Medicine, basil is warm and pungent. It helps circulate blood, promotes energy, and positively influences the spleen, stomach, lungs, and large intestine. Basil is excellent for digestion and effectively treats indigestion and stomach ache. It's also used to regulate menstruation. It has strong antibacterial properties and is very high in vitamin K. It contains eugenol, which inhibits an enzyme called cyclooxygenase (COX). This is exactly what many over-the-counter non-steroidal anti-inflammatory medications (NSAIDS) do. Therefore, basil can reduce inflammation and relieve symptoms of arthritis or inflammatory bowel conditions.

Chiffonade style of cutting

basil: Used to prepare fresh basil leaves. Arrange the flat whole basil leaves in a stack, roll the stack into a cigar shape, and slice thinly across the roll. Preserves the flavor, texture, and freshness of the herb.

Beef

In Traditional Chinese Medicine, beef has a neutral temperature and is sweet, affecting the spleen and stomach. It helps build blood and is therefore great for people with iron-deficiency anemia. Animal organ meats may affect the corresponding human organ. For example, beef liver supports the human liver, sharpening vision and aiding in detoxification. Beef kidney nourishes the human kidneys and improves sexual capacity. Always choose free-range and pastured (grass-fed) beef whenever possible, preferably locally raised. Some meat labeled "all natural" is actually grain-fed rather than grass-fed.

Beets

In Traditional Chinese Medicine, beets are neutral in temperature and sweet in flavor. They help improve circulation and purify the blood. They strengthen the heart, benefit the liver, moisten the intestines in cases of constipation, and can promote menstruation. Beets are a root vegetable and may help calm the spirit when feeling ungrounded and anxious. They've been shown to protect against coronary artery disease and stroke and to lower cholesterol. They are a great source of folates, and the top greens are an excellent source of carotenoids, flavonoid antioxidants, and vitamin A. Golden beets are sweet in flavor, strengthen the heart, relax the spirit, improve circulation, benefit the liver and spleen, moisten the intestines, and

when any colored beet is combined with carrots, help regulate hormones. Beets contain the phytochemical known as glycine betaine, which lowers blood homocysteine levels.

Broccoli

In Traditional Chinese Medicine, broccoli is cooling in nature, pungent, and slightly bitter. It affects the liver and gallbladder. Due to its goitrogenic properties, it should not be eaten raw by people with thyroid challenges or low iodine. (*Goitrogenic* means it impacts the functioning of your thyroid and actually turns it off for several hours after consumption.) It contains high amounts of vitamin C, sulfur, iron, and B vitamins, pantothenic acid, and vitamin A. Broccoli contains high levels of indol-3-carbinol (I3C), a food compound shown to reduce "bad estrogens," and di-indolyl-methane (DIM), which enhances estrogen elimination and a healthy testosterone/estrogen ratio. It is a "manly" food that supports healthy testosterone levels, yet it also helps women rid their bodies of accumulated fake estrogens from plastics. Broccoli is a cruciferous vegetable, and thus has excellent anti-cancer properties. According to researchers at Ohio

State University, a substance is produced when eating broccoli and Brussels sprouts that can block the proliferation of cancer cells. The laboratory and animal study discovered a connection between I3C and a molecule called Cdc25A, which is essential for cell division and proliferation. The research shows that I3C causes the destruction of that molecule and thereby blocks the growth of breast cancer cells.

Brussels Sprouts

In Traditional Chinese Medicine, Brussels sprouts have a warming nature, are sweet and bitter in taste, and positively influence the heart, small intestine, spleen, and stomach. These cruciferous veggies support digestion and are known for their anti-cancer properties. Like broccoli, they contain DIM, which is known to modulate immune function and is antiviral and antibacterial. DIM also helps clear unhealthy stores of estrogen in estrogen-dominant people. Brussels sprouts are an excellent source of vitamins C, A, and K, and important minerals such as copper, calcium, potassium, manganese, phosphorus, and iron. They also contain a glucoside called sinigrin, which appears to protect humans from colon cancer. They have been shown to decrease cholesterol and are a wonderful addition to a healthful eating plan.

Burdock

Burdock root is bitter, so you may wish to start small. Burdock is excellent for liver detoxification and is very dense in nutrients. It purifies the blood, aids in detoxification of the liver, prevents infections, acts as an antifungal and antimicrobial as well as a diuretic, and is excellent for skin problems such as eczema, psoriasis, acne, boils, and carbuncles. It provides powerful antioxidants, such as vitamin C, which fight the free radicals that damage cells and make us age more quickly. It is high in inulin, a natural dietary fiber that stimulates gut-friendly *Bifidobacteria*.

Butternut Squash

Winter squash, such as butternut, pumpkin, and acorn, is full of carotenoids such as alpha-carotene and beta-carotene, plus lutein, zeaxanthin, and beta-cryptoxanthin. We often think of winter squash as having high carbohydrate content; however, many of butternut squash's carbs come from polysaccharides and include special chains of D-galacturonic acid called homogalacturonan, which have antioxidant, anti-inflammatory, anti-diabetic, and insulin-regulating properties.

Winter squash also contains cucurbitacin molecules that are glycosides. As a part of the plant's natural survival mechanism, they are mildly toxic and taste bitter to animals, including humans. However, they are antiviral, antibacterial, and anti-inflammatory.

Cabbage

In Traditional Chinese Medicine, purple cabbage is slightly warming, sweet, and pungent. It improves digestion, benefits the stomach, and moistens the intestines. It's commonly used to treat whooping cough, constipation, and in conjunction with garlic, to expel worms from the intestines. It's high in sulfur and helps treat stomach and duodenal ulcers. People with thyroid challenges should avoid excessive amounts of raw cabbage because it is goitrogenic, unless it has been fermented in kimchi or sauerkraut. Cooked cabbage does not present this problem.

Chinese cabbage can help relieve constipation by affecting both the stomach and intestines. It decreases inflammation, benefits the kidneys, and can alleviate difficult burning urination.

Cacao/Chocolate (Raw)

Cacao contains theobromine, a stimulating caffeine-like chemical, and oxalic acid, which should be avoided by people with kidney stones and gout; however, it can also be used as a medicine and for ceremony and celebration. Its bitter flavor opens the heart and helps the liver. It raises dopamine and serotonin levels. It's an excellent source of magnesium, and therefore wonderful for heart health, muscle tension, menstrual cramps, and sluggish brain. It's also known for its aphrodisiac properties and is thus a powerful, sensual medicine.

Consult your healthcare provider to determine whether raw cacao—chocolate—can be part of your gut repair program. It comes from a bean but is also loaded with antioxidants. If you've done Cyrex Array 4 and have cross-reactivity to chocolate, remember that the chocolate used for that test is milk chocolate and what we are using here is raw cacao with no dairy whatsoever. There are still certain people who may react. Even I do at times. Raw cacao can help wean a person over to a strict gut-repair program or can be used after they've completed a comprehensive repair.

Cardamom

In India, cardamom is used medicinally as an anti-inflammatory and to treat symptoms of bladder infection, nephritis, and cystitis. It inhibits the growth of certain viruses, bacteria, and fungi, stimulates digestion, and increases the production of bile while relieving flatulence.

Carrots

In Traditional Chinese Medicine, carrots are neutral in temperature, sweet in flavor, and help direct *qi*, or life force energy, downward (the downward direction can be beneficial for coughs). Carrot soup can be used to treat whooping cough in children.

Carrots benefit the lungs, spleen, pancreas, stomach, and liver in several ways: they relieve excess stomach acid, can eliminate putrefaction of bacteria in the intestines, and can be used to treat diarrhea and chronic dysentery. They are high in silica, and therefore help rebuild connective tissue and bones. Carrots are also a diuretic and can help promote urination. Eating carrots with beef or chicken liver can help your liver and your vision.

Carrots relieve excess stomach acid; help dissolve accumulations, such as stones and tumors; and are alkalizing, thus treating symptoms such as acne, tonsillitis, urinary tract infections, and rheumatism. They help increase milk supply in nursing mothers and regulate hormones. The juice can be used topically to treat mild burns. They are rich in antioxidants such as beta-carotene, used to treat night blindness, other visual challenges, and ear infections. Many studies show that carrots decrease the risk of cardiovascular disease and certain types of cancers, such as colon.

It's better to eat them raw, baked, steamed, or stir-fried rather than boiled for both flavor and nutrient content. There are a wide variety of carrot colors (yellow, purple, red) that contain varying amounts of anthocyanindins, cancer-protecting antioxidants, so mix them up a bit and enjoy a wider variety of phyto (plant) nutrients.

Carrot Tops

Carrot tops are slightly bitter, high in chlorophyll, and an excellent source of magnesium, potassium, calcium, and vitamin K (important for bone health). I love to use them in pesto!

Cauliflower

Although typically it's a white vegetable (there are orange and purple varieties), cauliflower is still dense in nutrients. It contains sulforaphane and plant sterols, such as indole-3-carbinol (I3C) and di-indolyl-methane (DIM), which is an immune system modulator. It is high in fiber, and raw cauliflower contains high concentrations of vitamin C, manganese, potassium, and vitamins B1, B5, and B6. Cauliflower aids in detoxification, and contains glucosinolates, which can help activate detoxification enzymes and regulate their activity.

Celery

In Traditional Chinese Medicine, celery is cooling, sweet, and bitter. It benefits the stomach, spleen, and pancreas, and calms the liver. It improves digestion, dries excess dampness in the body, promotes sweating, and increases sperm count in men. It is high in silicon, and therefore great for connective tissue, bones, joints, and arteries. Eight ounces (240 ml) of celery juice for 10 consecutive days can greatly reduce uric acid levels in people predisposed to or experiencing gout. Both the stalks and root are used in the East and West to treat high blood pressure, even during pregnancy.

Celeriac (Celery Root)

Celeriac, or celery root, is a different plant from celery, despite its name and mild celery flavor. It is specially grown for its root and looks like a brownish alien hairball in the produce section of your local grocer.

It has a starchy potato-like texture like a turnip, but it contains little starch compared to other root veggies. It can be eaten raw or cooked. It is a fall and winter root but can often be found in local grocery stores, health food stores, and Asian markets year round.

Celeriac is an excellent addition to a gut-repair diet as it helps with many digestive problems, such as indigestion, ulcers, gastritis, and lack of appetite. It can also support healthy liver and bladder function. It helps alleviate swelling in cases of arthritis pain and digestive inflammation, and it can stimulate metabolism by quickening the fat-burning process. Historically, it was known as a natural aphrodisiac and was also used to improve endurance and treat people in a weakened or fragile state. It is rich in vitamins A, C, K, and E, carotene, and other micronutrients.

Cherries

Sour cherries benefit the liver, eyes, joints, and blood. These antioxidant-rich fruits may counter free-radical damage with few calories. We've learned from science that cherries contain *anthocyanins*, which act like anti-inflammatory agents by blocking the actions of cyclooxygenase-1 and -2 enzymes. This means they can help with painful episodes of gout by helping the body clear high levels of uric acid. They are rich in the stable antioxidant melatonin, thus supporting breast health, insomnia, and headaches, and quieting nervous system irritability.

Chia Seeds

In Traditional Chinese Medicine, chia seeds tonify *qi* and lubricate dryness. They are higher in omega-3 essential fatty acids than flax seeds and are a brain and body superfood! They've been traditionally used by Native Americans in the Southwest and South Americans for endurance and strength. They treat the symptoms of constipation and are just about the only seed that is safe during gut repair. They have high fiber content, which helps prevent sugar spikes. They are also high in phosphorus, protein, and calcium. When soaked, they become gelatinous, serving as a binder for raw foods, and for nut-free, egg-free, and grain-free cooking.

Chicken

In Traditional Chinese Medicine, chicken is warming and sweet. It tonifies *qi* and supports digestion. It can be used to treat spleen and pancreas imbalances that result in poor appetite, anorexia, low weight,

diabetes, diarrhea, edema, and weakness after childbirth. Don't shy away from organ meats. If your chicken comes with them, consider boiling them or leaving them in the crockpot to cook. Chicken liver can strengthen both the liver and kidneys and helps with childhood malnutrition, impotency, vision challenges, and certain types of anemia. Make certain to purchase organic, free-range birds whenever possible.

Cilantro (Coriander)

This leafy herb helps to naturally detoxify the body from heavy metals such as mercury. It contains healthy amounts of vitamins A, C, and K, plus phenolic flavonoid antioxidants such as quercetin, which is a bronchial dilator. It reduces allergic histamine reactions, is strongly anti-inflammatory, and may protect from certain types of cancers. It's used to treat conditions of the heart and blood vessels, such as high cholesterol and atherosclerosis (hardening of the arteries).

Cinnamon

In Traditional Chinese Medicine, cinnamon is pungent and slightly bitter in flavor and warming in thermal nature. It has anti-clotting properties and helps invigorate the blood. It also has been shown to lower

LDL (bad) cholesterol and help regulate blood sugar. Its odor can boost memory and cognitive function. Use with caution during pregnancy.

Cloves

This spice has antimicrobial, antifungal, antiseptic, antiviral, aphrodisiac, and stimulating properties. It has a cooling, anti-inflammatory effect on the lungs for cough and bronchitis, and for skin problems such as eczema and acne. It is commonly used for dental inflammation and pain, including teething.

Coconut

In Traditional Chinese Medicine, coconut is warming in nature, sweet, and strengthening to the heart and brain. It's an excellent source of good saturated fat. A diet high in good fats (a ketogenic diet), low to moderate protein, and no carbohydrates (other than veggies) is thought to improve brain function by 25 percent and is helpful in the treatment of epilepsy, heart disease, high blood pressure, traumatic brain injury, ADD/ADHD, autism, Asperger's, and Alzheimer's. Coconut butter is warm, sweet in flavor, and nourishing to yin. The Thai section of your grocery store may carry canned full-fat, organic coconut milk. Make sure it isn't thickened with wheat flour, which occurs in many Thai restaurants.

Coconut Aminos

This soy sauce alternative is made from raw organic coconut sap and is very tasty as a savory seasoning. It's free of gluten, dairy, and soy, has a very low glycemic index, and provides 17 amino acids, minerals, and vitamins.

Cooking tip: Best to add it to a stir-fry after it's been cooked to maintain the integrity of the amino acids.

Collard Greens

These leafy greens come from the cabbage family. If you have low thyroid, avoid consuming collards raw because they can decrease thyroid function. They're an excellent source of bioavailable calcium—much better than dairy products—and of other minerals, such as selenium and zinc. These gorgeous green leaves contain both soluble and insoluble fiber, which can help control LDL (bad) cholesterol and relieve constipation. They contain di-indolyl-methane (DIM) and sulforaphane, which provide benefits against breast, colon, prostate, and ovarian cancers. They're an excellent source of folates, vitamin A, carotenoids (antioxidants), vitamin C, and vitamin K—all very important for bone health and promoting osteotropic activity (that is, nourishing bone, or osseous, tissue).

Cranberries

In Traditional Chinese Medicine, cranberries support the water element, affecting the bladder and kidneys. They are sour and sweet in flavor, thereby supporting the liver, spleen, and stomach. They're wonderful for treating symptoms of urinary tract infections, although most commercial brands add sugar to juices and dried fruits and should be avoided during times of infection. Organic is best, not from concentrate, unfiltered, with no sugar or other fruit juices added. You can make your own dried cranberries. In a pinch, I have found some sweetened with organic apple juice.

Dandelion

Like mustard greens, dandelion greens support the liver and purify the blood. Bitter dandelion greens also support digestion, blood circulation, and aid in detoxification of the liver. Their bitterness comes from the crystalline compound taraxacin, which is therapeutic. Dandelion contains many beneficial flavonoids and is a good source of minerals. It's very low-calorie and acts as a laxative. It appears

to be the richest plant source of vitamin K, necessary for healthy bones and brains. It's also very high in vitamin A, an important antioxidant and fat-soluble vitamin necessary for healthy mucosa, skin, and eyes. Some coffee substitutes contain roasted dandelion root.

Fermented Foods

Fermented, or cultured, foods are raw, live foods that contain bacteria that are gut friendly and have been shown to aid in digestion, increase digestive enzymes, enhance immune function, help fend off harmful bacteria, and even fight cancer. They can also chelate—draw out—harmful toxins such as heavy metals. If you have high histamines, then fermented foods are likely not your friends.

Garlic

Garlic is naturally antifungal, antibacterial, and antiviral. It's excellent for treating symptoms of bronchitis and for urinary tract infections. It's known for its positive impact on the cardiovascular system. Raw is best for medicinal applications. Add it toward the end of your stir-fry. If you notice it causes you gas, then best to avoid for now.

Ginger

In Traditional Chinese Medicine, cold foods, such as ice cream, ice, cold drinks, tofu, milk, and raw foods like salads, can deplete the spleen energy and create dampness. Ever eaten ice cream and noticed a layer of mucus forming in your throat? Or your nose becomes stuffy? This is one symptom of dampness. Excess body fat is also viewed as a form of dampness. Dampness is better managed when the spleen is kept warm. Ginger warms the spleen and stomach, which improves digestion and decreases inflammation and dampness, thereby reducing mucus. It's known for its anti-inflammatory properties, but it must be consistently consumed for two months before chronic inflammation abates, so don't give up too soon.

Ginger makes a lovely tea. Simply peel and slice quarter-inch or 60 cm rounds of the root, and place them in a saucepan with water, bring to just under boiling on the stove and allow the mixture to simmer for 30 minutes.

Note: Do not boil, as boiling can ruin certain therapeutic properties.

Goji Berries

Goji berries, or wolfberries, are a power-packed superfruit from Asia. In Traditional Chinese Medicine, goji supports the liver and blood and nourishes the eyes and hair. These berries support the kidneys and can be useful in the treatment of low back pain due to kidney deficiency. They're in the nightshade family (*Solanaceae*), but most people gain great benefits from them, which is why I've included them as optional additions to several recipes. They have a high concentration of protein for a fruit and are very high in vitamin C. They also have strong antioxidant and anti-inflammatory properties and contain 21 trace minerals. They offer more iron than spinach.

You will find them most commonly in their dried form. The dried berries can be soaked, and the liquid added to teas, or you can simply drink the liquid. They can also be eaten alone or added to soups, smoothies, trail mix, or desserts.

Note: Before consuming these berries, check with your doctor if you are taking medications for diabetes or blood pressure, or the blood thinner Warfarin.

Hearts of Palm

Hearts of palm are rich in manganese, iron, potassium, and zinc, and contain about 4 grams of protein per cup (about 240 g or

240 ml). They even have vitamin B6. The majority of manganese in the human body is found in bones, with some in the kidneys, liver, pancreas, pituitary gland, and adrenal glands. Manganese may help prevent diabetes, heart disease, multiple sclerosis, osteoporosis, premenstrual syndrome, allergies, and rheumatoid arthritis. Manganese helps the body assimilate biotin, thiamin, ascorbic acid, and choline. It's beneficial in the synthesis of fatty acids and cholesterol, facilitates protein and carbohydrate metabolism, and may enable the production of sex hormones.

Hydrolyzed Yeast

Hydrolized yeast is code for monosodium glutamate (MSG), which should always be avoided. It may be present in store-bought vegetable or chicken broth and bouillon, so buyer beware! It is often also disguised as "natural flavoring".

Jerusalem Artichokes

Also known as sunchokes, these are a bit starchy but high in iron, vitamin C, phosphorus, potassium, and vitamin B1. They're also rich in inulin, a prebiotic, which promotes gut health by feeding friendly intestinal bacteria.

You can shred or dice them onto your salad or sauté thin slices with rosemary, sage, salt, and pepper to use as a potato substitute. They're starchy so use in moderation, depending upon which stage of gut repair you are in. If you're beginning a ketogenic diet or combating yeast and leaky gut, avoid for at least two months, unless they help you wean off white potatoes.

Kale

This cruciferous leafy vegetable is loaded with flavonoids and antioxidants and is naturally anti-inflammatory, helping to prevent chronic inflammatory diseases and oxidative stress. It's high in iron and calcium, and also contains vitamins K, A, and C, copper, sodium, potassium, manganese, and phosphorus. Steamed kale has been shown to reduce cholesterol. The vital nutrients in these greens are excellent for vision, bones, tendons, and ligaments, while supporting detoxification and cellular regeneration. Thanks to its detoxifying glucosinolate phytonutrients, kale has been shown to help in the treatment of colon and breast cancer and in the prevention of bladder, prostate, and ovarian cancers.

Note: Kale supports detoxification at the DNA level but is goitrogenic, which means it mildly inhibits thyroid function if eaten raw. Slightly steaming or cooking eliminates this effect.

Kefir

Kefir is a fermented yogurt-type drink containing many beneficial microorganisms. Check ingredients of whichever brand you buy; some contain tapioca inulin and may be cross-reactive. It's ideal to make your own, and it is superior to yogurt. It contains vitamins, minerals, amino acids, and enzymes. I encourage you to make it with coconut milk or water rather than dairy.

Note: Kefir grains may need a short time in an organic milk product to awaken their properties and then can go back into the coconut milk.

Kombucha

This fermented beverage smells like vinegar but tastes like a sparkling cider. It's been touted as a health elixir for at least 2,000 years, although there is little scientific research to date. It's said to prevent cancer and aid in detoxification of the liver, has anti-inflammatory properties, improves digestion, has B vitamins and antioxidants, and supports the immune function. If you have candida, avoid until you've fully resolved it. Some bodies don't do well

with it, so pay attention to how you feel.

Kudzu

This is a tuber from Japan that can be found in health food stores and Asian markets. It's been used to treat the symptoms of high blood pressure, insulin resistance, cardiovascular disease, menopause, and stomach ulcers, while soothing cravings for alcohol. It may inhibit the effects of estrogen therapy and antiarrhythmic agents and may lower blood sugar. It usually comes in small white chunks that need to be dissolved in a tiny bit of water before using.

Lamb

In Traditional Chinese Medicine, lamb is warming in nature, sweet in flavor, and affects the spleen and kidneys. It's a tonic that builds kidney strength. And in Oriental medicine, whenever you hear "tonify kidneys," think good sex! Yes, lamb can strengthen libido and erections. It's excellent for underweight people with weak constitutions, but should be eaten more moderately if you have heat in your body, a tendency toward high cholesterol due to fat metabolism impairments, or gallbladder problems.

Lemon

Lemon is astringent and sour. It supports the liver and gallbladder, reduces mucus, and is alkalizing, not acidic, to the body. It is very high in vitamin C, a water-soluble antioxidant that helps scavenge the damaging free radicals that cause us to age. It has anti-inflammatory properties and can assist in modulating (regulating, balancing) immune system function. It has antiseptic and antimicrobial properties as well.

Note: It's nice to add to water, but not daily as it can slowly wear away tooth enamel.

Limes

In Traditional Chinese Medicine, limes are sour, support liver function, and are alkalizing to the body. They assist in the digestion of fats, cleanse the blood, and help with cramps and sore throat. Limes are antiseptic, antimicrobial, and help resolve mucus. The zest of the lime supports the liver, decreases phlegm, and stimulates the digestion of fats.

Meats

Charbroiling, smoking, and barbecuing meats introduces a group of carcinogens (cancer-causing agents) called *nitrites* and *nitrosamines*. Studies suggest that red meat, especially those with higher fat content such as lamb and pork, have higher levels of nitrosamines. It's best to limit consumption of these kinds of foods. White meat has little to none.

Cooking tips: To enjoy a safe summer cookout on the grill, precook your meat in the oven and then finish it on the grill so it has a grilled flavor but fewer potentially hazardous toxins. Avoid charring or flame flare-ups by watching your grill closely and not grilling fatty meats that tend to drip down on the hot coals and create smoke, which carries the toxic nitrosamines back up into your food. Also avoid sugary marinades, which are more likely to burn, and make sure the charcoal is hot before beginning to grill the food to decrease the length of exposure. Using a marinade first helps protect the food.

Mustard Greens

Like dandelion greens, mustard greens support the liver and purify the blood. Their bitter, spicy flavor supports digestion and cardiovascular health. They are very high in vitamin K, folates, vitamins A and C, and are rich in antioxidants, flavonoids, indoles, sulforaphane, carotenes, lutein, and zeaxanthin, which can inhibit growth of certain cancers, such as prostate, colon, breast, and ovarian. They contain essential minerals necessary for maintaining health.

Olives

Olives contain healthy fats that nourish your hair, skin, nails, and brain.

Onions

Onions are pungent. They influence the lungs, reduce clotting, expel cold, and support protein metabolism. They are rich in chromium, which helps reduce and balance blood sugar levels in diabetics. They reduce cholesterol, are anti-cancer, antifungal, antibacterial, and antiviral. They contain an antioxidant flavonoid called *quercetin*, which is anti-inflammatory and anti-cancer as well.

Oregano

This herb is known for its essential oil carvacrol, which has potent antiviral, antibacterial, antifungal, antiseptic, and anti-spasmodic properties. It's used to treat colds and flus, upset stomach, mild fevers, herpes virus, and menstrual cramps. It facilitates gastro-intestinal enzyme secretion, stimulates digestion, and improves gut-motility (bowel movements). Like thyme, it is rich in antioxidant properties

and is high in vitamins K and A, iron, and manganese.

Parsnips

In Traditional Chinese Medicine, parsnips are warming and sweet. They benefit the spleen, pancreas, and stomach; can help clear the liver and gallbladder; are a mild diuretic; and lubricate the intestines. Parsnips provide fiber and are high in vitamins C, A, and E—antioxidants that are essential for tissue repair. They're a great source of folate, which helps prevent megaloblastic anemia (especially prevalent in vegetarians) and certain types of autoimmune disorders. Folate can also help lower blood homocysteine levels. Parsnips provide about 80 percent of the daily requirement for copper.

Peaches

In Traditional Chinese Medicine, peaches moisten yin—fluids in the body—and address symptoms such as a dry cough. Peaches are cooling, and their flavor is sweet, sour, and slightly astringent. When cooked and puréed, they can help with symptoms of gastrointestinal inflammation. TCM places great emphasis on the spleen's health—as gauged through the pulses—which is considered a marker of general health. Peach chutney warms the spleen with ginger, chili (but omit for strict gut repair), and pickling spices, which include clove, pepper, and cinnamon.

Pears

In Traditional Chinese Medicine, pears are cooling in thermal nature and sweet and slightly sour in flavor. They eliminate heat and excess mucus in the lungs. They also moisten the lungs and throat, quench thirst, and reduce inflammation. They can be used to treat certain heat symptoms associated with diabetes, skin challenges, constipation, and gallbladder obstruction.

Pomegranates

These beautiful fruits are very high in antioxidants and therefore help repair DNA, thus preventing or slowing certain types of cancer, such as prostate. They have been shown to improve blood flow to the heart in people with coronary heart disease. Certain compounds found in the juice may help reduce the risk of heart disease. They may inhibit the build-up of plaque in the blood vessels. According to cardiac specialist Dr. Dean Ornish (see *www.nutrition-and-you.com /pomegranate.html*), "Certain ellagitannin compounds, such as granatin B and punicalagin found in the juice, are effective in reducing the risk of heart

disease by scavenging harmful free radicals. Some research suggests that they stop the build-up of plaque in the blood vessels."

Protein Powder

Not all protein powders are created equally. If it lists things you can't pronounce or has synthetic flavors or vitamins, then don't buy it. Avoid whey protein concentrate powders if you have a sensitivity to lactalbumin. Whey hydrolysate is easier to digest. Free-range beef protein isolates, organic pea protein, collagen hydrolysate, concentrated bone broth isolate, or bovine serum albumin protein are great options. Be careful of hemp protein, unless you've done Cyrex Array 4 and know you don't cross-react to it.

Pumpkin

In Traditional Chinese Medicine, pumpkin is cooling in thermal nature and sweet and slightly bitter in flavor. Warming spices such as cinnamon help to balance its cooling nature. It's been used in the treatment of diabetes symptoms and hypoglycemia, helps regulate blood sugar, benefits the pancreas, and relieves damp conditions such as edema and even bronchial asthma. It's high in vitamins C and A, plus leutin and zeaxanthin, all of which may help prevent symptoms of cataracts and improve macular degeneration.

Radishes

Radishes are small, pungent, and spicy cruciferous root vegetables that promote digestion and help alleviate abdominal distention due to sluggish digestion. In Traditional Chinese Medicine, they are used to support overall detoxification and to help cool lung conditions associated with heat, such as cough with yellow mucus. The black radishes are spicier. The watermelon radishes are beautifully colored and a little sweeter. They are high in vitamin C and antioxidants and contain sulforaphane, which protects against certain types of cancers. Save the green tops for stir-fries and soups.

Salmon

This fish is loaded with healthy omega-3 fatty acids in the form of EPA (eicosapentaenoic acid) and a slightly lower amount in the form of DHA (docosahexaenoic acid). Omega-3s can help prevent blood clots and decrease the risk of stroke. Salmon has a very beneficial omega-3 to omega-6 ratio. These fish oils are most abundant in brain cells, nerve relay stations, retinas, adrenal glands, and sex glands. DHA is one of the most important fats for your brain. Eating salmon can positively impact cognitive faculties and improve mood. The omega-3s have also been shown to protect joints, possibly prevent macular degeneration, and support healthy vision. Salmon is high in the mineral selenium, an important antioxidant that protects the cardiovascular system, decreases risk of joint inflammation, prevents certain types of cancer, and aids in proper thyroid function. It's also a good source of protein that is easy to digest. It provides B vitamins, vitamin D, and even tryptophan. Salmon may help prevent Parkinson's and Alzheimer's diseases.

Note: Avoid farmed fish, as they are fed unnatural food and swim in their own waste. Wild Alaska salmon are considered the most healthful to eat, but use caution about eating Pacific fish at this time as it may be contaminated by radiation poisoning following the Fukushima nuclear accident in Japan. Salmon is excellent. Do your best to get wild salmon. If you simply cannot, then eat in moderation, and consider eating wild sardines.

Sardines

Like salmon, sardines are full of important omega-3 fatty acids, which support heart and brain health. Sardines provide many of the same health benefits as salmon. I always purchase them with the bone for added bioavailable calcium.

Spinach

In Traditional Chinese Medicine, spinach is cooling in thermal nature and sweet in flavor. It supports both the large and small intestines, cleanses the blood, and is used to treat skin disorders that are hot (red) and itchy. It lubricates dryness and helps relieve constipation, symptoms of hemorrhoids, nose bleeds, hypertension (high blood pressure), headaches, and even dizziness in certain circumstances. Spinach is high in antioxidants, anti-inflammatory, and anti-cancer, especially prostate cancer. The more vibrantly green it is, the more nourishing it is. It's packed with vitamins K and A, manganese, folate, and iron. Vitamin K is necessary for bone health.

Note: Spinach contains oxalates and may exacerbate kidney or gallbladder problems (such as stones), as oxalates can impair iron and calcium absorption. It's also high in purines and should be avoided by people with gout. Enjoy it raw, boiled (dispose of the water due to its acid content), and stir-fried,

but be sure to consume kale and collards for more calcium. Spinach contains glycoglycerolipids, which are the main fat-related molecules in the membranes of light-sensitive organs in most plants and are therefore indispensable for plant photosynthesis. Recent research in laboratory animals shows that glycoglycerolipids from spinach can help protect the lining of the digestive tract from damage, especially damage related to unwanted inflammation.

Strawberries

According to Traditional Chinese Medicine, strawberries are cooling in nature and sweet and sour. They can relieve indigestion, sore throat, hoarseness, and thirst, and can help eliminate symptoms of gout. They are high in vitamin C, anthocyanins, and ellagic acid that are known to be anti-cancer, anti-aging, and anti-inflammatory. They also contain important B-complex vitamins.

Note: Always purchase organic berries, and wash them well. All of those tiny seed indentions soak up pesticides and herbicides, making soft berries among the most contaminated items on the annual Dirty Dozen list of produce.

Sweet Potatoes

In Traditional Chinese Medicine, sweet potatoes are neutral in temperature and sweet. They support the stomach, spleen, and kidneys, especially as a yin tonic. Fluids of the body are yin, so sweet potatoes can be useful when someone feels dry, or has premature ejaculation. Sweet potatoes are rich in antioxidants. They contain vitamins C, A, and E; lots of beta-carotene (a precursor to vitamin A); and magnesium, iron, calcium, and potassium. This combination makes sweet potatoes a beauty food since vitamins C and E and beta-carotene all play essential roles in nurturing glowing skin and strong thick hair. They're also high in vitamin B6, which can help reduce the toxic amino acid homocysteine, which is linked to cardiovascular and other degenerative diseases. Sweet potatoes do not need to be cooked, but they are starchy, so enjoy in moderation.

Tarragon

This is one of the four main herbs used in French cooking. It also has antioxidant properties, acting as a free-radical scavenger. It has a high content of eugenol, similar to the oil found in cloves, which has a numbing effect when chewed and has often been used for toothache. It's a good source of potassium and supports digestion by aiding in bile production, helping to alleviate dyspepsia and irritable bowel, while stimulating the appetite. It can help promote sleep.

Note: It's known for promoting delayed menstruation and should be avoided during pregnancy.

Thyme

This herb contains thymol, a very healing essential oil that is antiseptic and antifungal. It's known to have the highest antioxidant value of any herb, containing many flavonoid phenolic antioxidants, such as lutein, thymonin, pigenin, zeaxanthin, and naringenin. It contains B6 (pyridoxine), vitamin C, vitamin A, beta-carotene, vitamin K, vitamin E, and folic acid.

Tuna

Tuna is a larger fish and therefore tends to accumulate mercury, so it is wise to limit consumption. Always purchase wild tuna. Avoid bluefin tuna, since they are the largest, longest-lived, and most endangered tuna species. Tongol, yellowfin, and albacore are better choices. Tuna is high in omega-3 fatty acids; it is therefore great for cardiovascular health, eyes, hair, and brain, and acts as an anti-inflammatory.

Turmeric

This rhizome, which is related to ginger, is a strong anti-inflammatory that helps halt autoimmune flare-ups, especially when combined with resveratrol. Curcumin, the principal pigment of this root, is known for its anti-tumor, antioxidant, anti-arthritic, anti-amyloid (amyloid is the protein suspected to cause brain degeneration in Alzheimer patients), anti-ischemic (protects against heart attack), anti-flatulent, antimicrobial, and anti-inflammatory properties. Its rich orange color stains, so wear an apron. It's been used to dye Easter eggs and fabric. I peel the root and then dice it for soups and stir-fries.

Note: Use with extreme caution in cases of high blood pressure being treated with medication, as it can dramatically drop blood pressure and therefore requires close monitoring and possibly alteration of prescription drug use.

Vinegar

In Traditional Chinese Medicine, vinegar is warming and moves stagnant blood. The sour and bitter flavors reduce liver accumulations. It can be used as a foot bath for symptoms of athlete's foot fungus. It relieves damp conditions such as excess mucus and edema, and stops bleeding. Apple cider vinegar can be taken prior to each meal to support healthy digestion and absorption of vital nutrients. It's commonly used in bone broth to extract nutrients from the bone marrow.

Chapter 18

Recipes

E ach of the primary recipes that follows is 100 percent gut repair-friendly. Some variations and options are not conducive to gut repair, and I have noted them as such. I include them in this book to give your friends and family options and give you more choices to explore once your gut is fully repaired and you have no autoimmune challenges or other sensitivities that have been identified.

Please assume that all ingredients listed are organic. Do your best to shop for locally grown and seasonal foods. All meat should be pastured (grass-fed), organic, and happy. All fish should be wild.

Substitute your favorite veggies in any recipe, but know that I chose particular ingredients for their combined therapeutic properties, taste, and color. Enjoy the creative process on your sumptuous journey of self-love and healthy eating!

Note: I sometimes list non-keto ingredients as a separate option. These can be included if you're having guests and want to "dress up" a recipe or are opening your diet back up to include more foods. Please follow my suggestions when it comes to these "optional" ingredients. In addition, some recipes include ingredients that are higher in carbohydrates, such as parsnips and sweet potato. These are transitional recipes, noted as such, that are designed for people slowly moving toward a ketogenic diet or who have severe adrenal fatigue and require more carbohydrate during their healing. You can eat *some* of them if you're strictly keto—just not too much! If you have Crohn's disease it is important to avoid all seeds and nuts at this time, so skip recipes that contain ingredients such as chia, flax, pepitas.

Bon appétit!

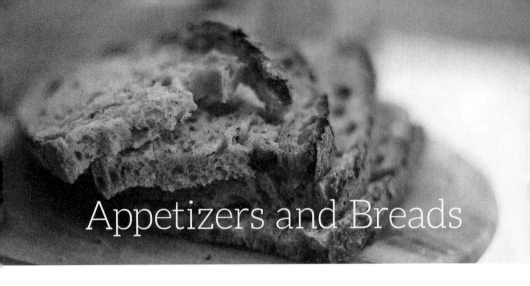

Appetizers and Breads

Spicy Thai Collard Wraps

This was a favorite recipe even before I learned about gut repair. The presentation is beautiful, and the eating is finger-dripping-licking good! If you have low thyroid, avoid consuming collards raw, because they can decrease thyroid function; you need not worry here, however, because the collards are blanched.

Ingredients

6–8 large collard leaves (will yield 12–16 wraps)

3 Tbsp umeboshi plum vinegar or coconut vinegar

3–4 Tbsp olive oil

1 clove (or to taste) garlic, pressed or minced

2–3 Tbsp ginger, peeled and finely shredded or minced (grated ginger can be stringy, so just discard that last stringy chunk)

½ cup/75 g green onions, finely chopped, including the green stalks

1–2 kaffir lime leaves, sliced very thin (optional); I use about a Tbsp of pre-cut leaves in a jar with citric acid

¼ cup/60 ml lime juice

1½ Tbsp coconut aminos

1 large organic carrot or 1 cup/ 150 g baby carrots, grated or cut into matchsticks (baby carrots are easier to cut)

1 small jicama root, peeled and cut into matchsticks (jicama roots are often large, so I ask the produce manager to cut one in half for me)

1 small cucumber, cut into matchsticks (don't try to grate this in a food processor—it's too watery!)

½ cup/20 g packed fresh mint leaves

20 fresh basil leaves

Options (okay for gut repair)

4–5 very thin stalks of raw organic asparagus, cut into 1–2-inch (2.5–5 cm) pieces; asparagus should be consumed within 2 days of purchase, or wrap the ends in a moistened paper towel to preserve freshness

2 cups/200 g mung bean sprouts, or other sprouts of your liking

Options (not for gut repair, but nice for guests or potlucks)

3 Tbsp unrefined sesame oil, for the sauce

3 heaping Tbsp raw almond butter, (smooth not crunchy is best) for the sauce (may add after 2 months of gut repair)

1 mango or papaya, peeled, seeded, and cut into ¼-inch or 50 cm strips, to garnish the tops of the wraps

Preparation

- Bring a large pot of water to a simmering boil. Submerge the collard leaves in boiling water for about 10 seconds. Remove them with tongs, and submerge into a large bowl of ice water. This halts the cooking process and keeps their vibrant green color. Set them aside to cool.
- In a bowl, mix together the oil, optional almond butter or sesame oil, garlic, ginger, green onions, kaffir lime leaves, lime juice, remaining 2 Tbsp vinegar, coconut aminos, and sea salt to taste. **Note:** This can be made ahead of time and kept for 2 days in a sealed container in the fridge. It's delicious over chopped lettuce or spinach.
- Toss the carrots, jicama, cucumbers, mung bean sprouts (perhaps save some to garnish on top), and mint (perhaps save some to garnish) in the dressing. When the collard leaves are cold, gently squeeze and blot with a clean dry towel. Toss in a shallow bowl containing a mixture of 1 Tbsp of umeboshi plum vinegar until completely coated on both sides. Add more vinegar as needed.
- Lay out one collard leaf and, with a paring knife, cut out the middle stem/vein. Each collard leaf will yield two wraps. Make sure the back side of the leaf is facing you so that the greener side will form the exterior of the wrap.
- Scoop the veggie/dressing mixture onto a leaf, half at the end closest to you. Fold the end over the veggie mixture, add a basil leaf and then roll it up like a burrito, folding in the sides of the leaf.
- Top it with either a few strips of mango or papaya, a small bunch of mung bean sprouts, a few sprigs of cilantro, or a few mint leaves, then place a piece of basil over the top (or under the mango).
- Now they're ready to be gobbled up! Leftovers are great the next day— they seem even tastier when they've had time to marinate.

Coconut Chia Protein Bread

I have found many adaptations for this gluten-free bread,
including a thin pizza crust. Since it's leavened with baking
powder rather than yeast, it does not rise like bread, but more
like an American biscuit (scone). It will also remain somewhat
moist when the baking is complete. My husband said,
"It's cake, and the coconut butter on top is the icing!"
You just can't go wrong with this one.

Ingredients

1 cup/120 g coconut flour

½ cup/50 g protein powder

2 tsp baking powder,
aluminum-free

1 tsp baking soda (bicarbonate
of soda)

½ cup/90 g chia meal (ground
chia seeds). Do not use whole
seeds; you won't get the
desired result—I grind my own
in a coffee/herb grinder)

¼ tsp sea salt

1¼ cups/300 ml coconut milk,
warmed to room temperature

⅓ cup/70 g or 80 ml coconut oil,
melted

2 tsp apple cider vinegar (or
lemon juice)

Preparation

- Preheat oven to 325°F. Lightly coat a medium loaf pan (approx. 8 x 4
  x 3 inches or 20 x 10 x 8 cm) with coconut oil or use a stone loaf pan
  or muffin cups. Sift together the dry ingredients. Combine the wet
  ingredients, possibly heating the coconut oil until it is liquid. Add the
  dry mix to the wet mix, and combine well.
- Form the dough into a big ball. Let sit for about 5 minutes to help set
  the chia seeds.
- Place dough into loaf pan, and gently form to pan with rubber spatula.
- Bake for 40–55 minutes, depending on your oven and altitude. (In
  Flagstaff, Arizona, at 7,000 feet above sea level, it takes about 55
  minutes in a convection oven. At about 2,000 feet above sea level, it
  takes 40 minutes.) Do the toothpick test to see if it's done. (Insert a
  toothpick into the finished loaf, then remove. If dough sticks to the
  toothpick, then bake another 5–10 minutes and repeat the test.)

- I typically use a large loaf pan. It firms up nicely in the fridge. I enjoy it slightly chilled, while my husband prefers it warm and toasted in the toaster oven.
- Allow to cool prior to slicing, and top with your favorite coconut butter and blueberries—YUM! My husband prefers mixing a little coconut oil with coconut butter (aka coconut manna) to make it more spreadable. Works like a charm!

Variation: Muffins
- Press dough into muffin cups.
- Bake for 25 percent less time than for a loaf.

Variation: Pizza Crust
- Thinly spread dough onto a pizza stone and bake for about 30 minutes.
- Allow to cool and then add toppings—such as the Tomato-Free Marinara Sauce or Raw Pesto in this book—plus sliced zucchini/ courgettes, olives, turkey bacon, roasted chicken chunks, artichoke hearts, broccoli, and a drizzle of olive oil.
- Place on a lower rack, and bake again for 30 minutes, or until done. If the crust is browning too much, cover the edges with aluminum foil.

Raw Chia Seed Crackers

These crackers are as simple as it gets! In three easy steps, they're ready to go: soak, shape, and dehydrate. They're a great snack. You can add herbs to them, or keep them plain. Enjoy them with dips from this book, with coconut butter, or just on their own. Some people with ulcerative colitis may need to refrain from these seeds for several months of gut repair. After your gut is healed, you can branch out and add cashew nut butter.

Ingredients
1–2 cups/180–360 g organic chia seeds

1 tsp ground, rosemary, thyme, oregano, basil (all optional)

pink sea salt to taste

water—enough to almost float them

Options (not for gut repair)

½ cup/65 g sunflower seeds

½ cup/30 g pepitas
  (pumpkin seeds)

⅓ cup/20 g diced sun-dried
  tomatoes

Preparation

- Pour the chia seeds into a bowl, and add enough water to soak them, not float them. Soak 15–60 minutes, or overnight for convenience.
- Spread on parchment paper with a rubber spatula, in any size or shape you desire. Lay on dehydrator tray, and salt. They need to be relatively thin. (If you make them too thick it will take longer to dehydrate.)
- Dehydrate at 108°F for about 3 hours or overnight until crunchy. (If you don't own a dehydrator, you can also make these in the oven on the lowest possible temperature. Keep a close watch on them, as they may only need an hour.)

Keto Buns

This recipe is both grain- and egg-free, perfect for snacks or with meals. The buns can be shaped to be small dinner roll size or larger hamburger buns.

They contain healthy fats and no sugar. The nutmeal can be substituted for extra coconut flour, depending on where you are in your gut repair program. The mesquite flour (can be found online or in specialty stores) helps stabilize your blood sugar, and the psyllium husks will support intestinal detoxification. If you can't find mesquite, don't worry; you can increase your nutmeal or coconut flour.

I prefer them topped with ghee (lactose- and casein-free) and after gut repair, cashew nut butter. It satisfies any desire I ever may have for some kind of bread or dinner roll. I usually double this recipe and freeze them. This recipe can be either transitional or fully ketogenic.

Ingredients

1½ cups/180 g nutmeal flour
(I often use half hazelnut and
half Brazil nut). If on strict gut
repair, then substitute coconut
flour, tapioca flour (if you
don't cross-react), or sweet
potato flour.

½ cup/90 g ground chia seeds
(chia meal)

½ cup/90 g psyllium husks

⅓ cup/60 g ground flax seeds
(flax meal)

⅓ cup/40 g coconut flour

¼ cup/30 g mesquite flour

1½ tsp cinnamon

2 tsp cream of tartar

2 tsp baking soda (bicarbonate
of soda)

1 tsp liquid vanilla or powdered
vanilla (or scrape a vanilla
bean pod)

dash of sea salt

20 drops liquid stevia or to taste

2 cups/500 ml boiling water

Variations

You can use rosemary, thyme, sage, and oregano for a savory version.
If you don't have cream of tartar, use 2 Tbsp apple cider vinegar with
3 tsp baking powder.

Preparation

- Preheat oven to 350°F.
- Combine all dry ingredients first, and stir them well. Gradually add
  boiling water to the dry ingredients, and incorporate well. It will bubble
  a little. This is normal.
- Make sure all dry ingredients have touched the water and there
  isn't any powder left at the bottom of the bowl. Use a large spoon to
  integrate the dry ingredients with water.
- Begin making your keto buns with your hands. Be careful, as the
  mixture is still hot. I shape them into medium-sized, not perfectly
  round balls. For hamburger buns, shape them larger.
- Place buns on a baking tray about ½ inch or 50 cm apart (they won't
  spread out like cookies often do).
- Bake at 350°F for 40–50 minutes.
- Allow to cool on a baking tray.
- Serve warm with ghee; refrigerate or freeze for longer shelf life.

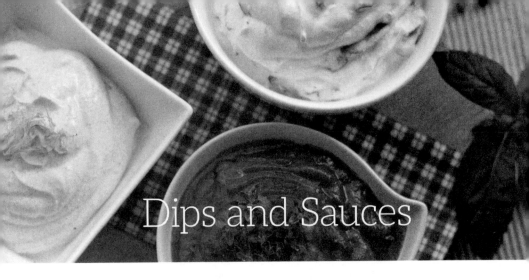

Dips and Sauces

Tomato-Free Marinara Sauce

Think you'd never be able to have marinara sauce on a
gut-repair diet? Think again! Here's a revised Italian classic
that will leave red splotches at the corners of your smile!
I like to pair this with yellow squash or zucchini noodles.

Ingredients

1 onion, diced (I like yellow or
white onions for this one)

1–2 Tbsp coconut oil

5 carrots, sliced

1–2 medium red beets, peeled
and diced into small chunks to
ensure faster cooking

**1½–2 cups/360–500 ml water,
chicken stock, or veggie stock**

2 garlic cloves, minced, or to taste

1 tsp parsley, dried

1 Tbsp basil, dried

1 tsp oregano, dried

½ tsp thyme, dried

½ tsp sea salt, or to taste

**1 tsp lemon juice, or apple cider
vinegar** (optional)

¼ tsp black pepper

Option (gut repair-friendly)
1 lb/500 g Italian sausage or ground turkey meat, sautéed, for the sauce

Option (not for gut repair)
½ cup/40 g button or shiitake mushrooms

Preparation

- Sauté the onions, garlic, and herbs, and optional mushrooms in
  coconut oil in a medium or large pan, preferably with a lid. Cook onions
  until soft, about 5–8 minutes. You may sauté the garlic cloves with the

onions, or for more kick, cook them less by adding them later along with the herbs.

- Add the carrots, beet chunks, and about ¾–1 cup/180–240 ml water. The finer you cut the beets, the faster they will cook.
- Cover and cook veggies over medium-low heat or at a simmer. Cook until the beets are soft, about 20–25 minutes. Check periodically to make sure there is still some water in the pan and they're not burning.
- When beets are cooked through, add about ½–1 cups/120–240 ml more water, salt, and pepper. Blend veggies with water until smooth. If your pan is deep enough, keep them there and use a hand blender, or transfer from the pot into a big blender. Add more water as necessary to achieve a marinara-like consistency. Add more herbs and/or salt to taste. If you would like some tang, add lemon juice or apple cider vinegar to make it more acidic, like tomato sauce.

This recipe makes a large batch that keeps well in the fridge for over a week. I use some for dinner the night I make it, then put half of the remaining sauce in a couple of containers and freeze for future meals.

I bake or steam spaghetti squash or stir-fry yellow squash noodles and add this sauce to create a gut repair-friendly pasta dinner. Create a bed of baby spinach, add the piping hot squash—which wilts the spinach—then top with marinara and meat. Delicioso! Italian gut repair dinner!

Cauli-Fredo Sauce

This sauce is amazing! It's perfect to add to
vegetables like broccoli or to baked chicken.

Ingredients

1 head of cauliflower, cored and chopped into large chunks

2 Tbsp avocado oil or refined coconut oil (largely free of coconut aroma and flavor)

1 shallot, minced

1 cup/240 ml chicken broth

¼ cup/60 ml canned coconut milk

salt and pepper to taste

Option (not for strict gut repair)

pinch of nutmeg

Preparation

- Steam cauliflower until fork-tender.
- While cauliflower steams, heat avocado oil or coconut oil in a small saucepan over medium-low heat. Add shallot and sauté for a few minutes, then add chicken broth and heat through.
- Place cauliflower, shallot/broth mixture, and remaining ingredients in a blender. Blend until smooth and creamy. Add more coconut milk if needed.
- Serve over ANYTHING, but tastes good on chicken and broccoli.

Keto Raw Pesto

This is a favorite of mine! When I eliminated nuts and seeds from my diet, I feared I might be unable to enjoy my beloved pesto, so I resolved to create a gut repair-friendly version. Our dear friends Steve and Lily taught me how to extend the shelf life of the basil by submerging the stems in a glass or bowl of water. No more wilty, brown basil! This versatile pesto can be used as a dip, a topping for chicken, or over baked spaghetti squash.

Ingredients

4 cups/240 g basil
½ cup/30 g parsley
1–2 cups/30–60 g baby spinach
1 avocado, pitted and peeled
2–3 cloves garlic

3–4 Tbsp olive oil
1 Tbsp lemon or lime juice, or juice from ½ large lemon or to taste
sea salt to taste

Options (okay for gut repair)
½ cup/15 g carrot tops or the tops of 1–2 carrots
½ cup/15 g arugula

½ cup/15 g dandelion greens or other wild greens such as purslane
¼ cup/60 ml coconut kefir

Options (not for gut repair)
1 Tbsp pumpkin seed oil
1 Tbsp macadamia nut oil
½ cup/30 g pepitas
½ cup/65 g sunflower seeds

½ cup/60 g pine nuts
½ cup/60 g walnuts
½ cup/60 g macadamia nuts
dash of pepper

Preparation

- Add all ingredients to food processor, and process into a paste. Clear the sides of the food processor often with a rubber spatula. If you need more liquid, you can add a Tbsp of water or oil, one at a time, until the desired consistency is achieved.
- Serve with raw zucchini pasta, baked spaghetti squash, or dehydrated zucchini chips, or use as a spread on raw collard wraps or dip with veggies or raw chia seed crackers. I make zucchini pasta with my spiral vegetable slicer (aka spiralizer); I love it!

Kristin's Famous Vegan Guacamole

Ketogenic diets require healthy fats. This snack is loaded with brain, skin, hair, and eye support. You can choose between the one creamy and two chunky guacamole variations presented here. Serve in a large bowl or spoon into half skins of avocados for a lovely presentation.

Ingredients

6 avocados, cut in half, pitted and scooped out of the skins (save the skins to use as serving dishes)

2–3 cloves garlic, diced

2 green onions, diced

½ cup/25 g chopped cilantro

1–2 red radishes, diced

1–2 limes, juiced

sea salt, to taste

Options (not for gut repair)

¾ cup/60 ml puréed macadamia nuts (about 1 cup/120 g macadamia nuts and ¼ cup/ 60 ml water, blended in food processor; add more water, if necessary, until thick and creamy)

1–2 tomatoes chopped (use in the guacamole or as a top garnish)

dash of cayenne or a diced jalapeño pepper or serrano chili (remove seeds for less kick)

black pepper to taste

Preparation: Creamy

- Place avocados in food processor with all other ingredients (omit tomatoes), and blend until smooth.

Preparation: Chunky
- Place half (3–4) of the avocados in food processor with all other ingredients except tomatoes, and blend until mostly smooth. Cube the remaining avocados and tomatoes, and gently stir in.

Preparation: Very Chunky
- You may avoid the food processor altogether and prepare everything with a knife. Cube all avocados and tomatoes, and stir well with the remaining ingredients.
- Garnish with sprigs of cilantro, chopped cilantro, tomato chunks, and a wedge of lime.
- Enjoy with veggies, raw seed crackers, sweet potato chips, lettuce wraps, on top a leafy green stir-fry, or raw kale chips.
- Serve immediately, or refrigerate and serve later. **Note:** If you aren't serving right away, make sure to save some of the avocado pits, and place them in the guacamole to keep it from turning brown too quickly.

Hearts of Palm Dip

Hearts of palm come from the core and bud of certain palm trees. Most are imported from Costa Rica. They're nice in stir-fries, gluten-free pizza, sauces, and dips.

Ingredients
1 can hearts of palm

3 Tbsp olive oil

1 tsp lemon juice

2 cloves garlic

3 Tbsp Italian parsley, chopped

sea salt to taste

Option (okay for gut repair)
1 avocado, for a creamier dip

Option (not for gut repair)
pepper to taste
dash of pepper or paprika, or spice it up with a dash of cayenne

Preparation
- Put all ingredients in a food processor, and blend until smooth.
- Serve with carrots, celery, and sliced cucumber. Makes about 1½ cups.

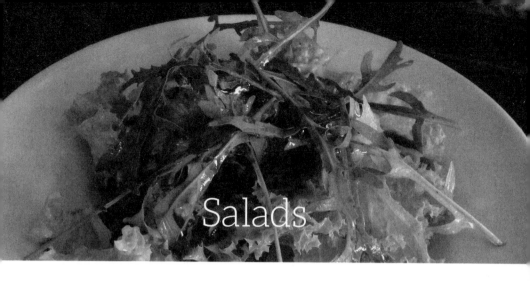

Salads

Asian Slaw with Dressing

This is a simple summer salad with Chinese cabbage, ginger, and Jerusalem artichokes/sunchokes.

Salad Ingredients

4 cups/360 g Chinese cabbage, leafy portion removed, remainder cut diagonally into ¼-inch-wide strips (or abut 50 cm); green or purple cabbage can also be used

1 carrot, cut into thin strips or shredded in food processor

1 cucumber, cut into thin strips

1 medium watermelon radish (or some other red radish), shredded or sliced in food processor

4 Tbsp chopped fresh cilantro

2 green onions, chopped

Salad Options (okay for gut repair)

several Jerusalem artichokes/sunchokes, washed and diced or grated

1 bulb fennel, chopped or grated in food processor

Salad Options (not for gut repair)

1 red bell pepper, seeded and cut into thin strips

1 tomato, chopped

Dressing Ingredients

¼ cup/60 ml olive oil

1 Tbsp lime juice

1 Tbsp coconut aminos or to taste

1–2 tsp grated/puréed fresh ginger

¼ cup/60 ml water, or coconut milk, or unsweetened coconut kefir, as needed for quantity and consistency

Dressing Option (okay for gut repair)
2½ tsp pumpkin seed oil, lends a unique flavor

Dressing Options (not for gut repair)
¼ cup/70 g gluten-free sweet white miso. **Note:** find one that has been fermented for 1–3 years rather than just a few weeks.
2½ tsp **Asian sesame oil** (possibly cross-reactive; Cyrex Array 4 will tell you if it's true for you.)

Preparation
- Whisk together dressing ingredients, and combine salad ingredients in a large bowl.
- Just before serving, add half the dressing to the salad and toss until vegetables are lightly coated. Add additional dressing as desired.
- Serve immediately, while fresh.

Arugula, Carrot, Golden Beet, and Ginger Salad with Cranberries

This spring salad is certain to satisfy all taste buds! In Traditional Chinese Medicine, it's important to eat with the season and for the season. This tasty salad is associated with spring but can be eaten any time.

Ingredients

1 or more bunches of arugula (rocket)
4 medium carrots, grated
1 large golden beet, grated
1½–2-inch/4–5 cm piece of peeled ginger root, grated or minced
¼–½ medium lemon, or to taste, juiced
2–5 Tbsp olive oil (as fresh and local as you can get)

2 Tbsp pomegranate balsamic vinegar or a specialty gourmet balsamic with floral or zesty flavor
2 Tbsp fresh basil, chopped chiffonade style (optional)
dash of pink sea salt and cracked ground pepper

Options (not for gut repair)

2–3 Tbsp pumpkin seed oil in addition to the olive oil

½ cup/80 g dried cranberries, no sulfur, unsweetened or sweetened with apple juice (depending on your level of gut repair and health challenges, this dried fruit, in small amounts in this recipe, might be just fine, consult your healthcare provider)

¼ cup/15 g pepitas (pumpkin seeds)

½–1 cup/75–150 g baby tomatoes

Preparation

- Grate the carrots and beets (I use the grater attachment on my food processor).
- Peel and mince or grate the ginger. The important thing is to avoid long, stringy fibers. If you use a grater, be sure to make a final pass with a knife to chop up any remaining long fibers.
- Toss everything else together in a bowl. Taste to see if you desire more vinegar, oil, lemon, or salt and pepper.
- Garnish with slices of avocado and serve!

Boogie for Brussels Sprouts

If you've never boogied for Brussels sprouts, this is the dish you've been waiting for! The first time I made it, I did a happy dance because it was so delicious and easy. I literally ran upstairs to my husband's office to give him a taste. He even asked what it was, being unable to identify the main ingredient. It reminds me of a warm cabbage slaw. You can serve it warm or cold, making it perfect for any season, although Brussels sprouts tend to be a winter crop.

Ingredients

½ lb/225 g turkey bacon (or pork bacon—not for gut repair), cooked and cut into small pieces; to make more protein-dense, add 1–2 more pieces

¼ cup/60 ml Dijon mustard (or stoneground, in which case use horseradish, see below)

2 Tbsp apple cider vinegar

3 Tbsp fresh lemon juice

¼ cup/60 ml avocado or coconut oil

2 lbs/1 kg Brussels sprouts, trimmed

2 green onions, cut on the bias

2–3 Tbsp pomegranate,
raspberry, or blackberry
ginger balsamic vinegar

3 Tbsp horseradish (use with
stoneground mustard—Dijon
already contains this ingredient,
unless you desire more "kick")

¼ tsp ground black pepper
sea salt to taste

Options (not for gut repair—about 2 months)

1–1½ cups/120–180 g large pecan halves, toasted (place pecans on small
rimmed baking sheet, and bake until toasted, stirring frequently, about
10–15 minutes; be careful not to burn them)

1 cup/100 g organic red grapes cut in half

Variations (not gut repair-friendly)

1 chopped or shredded Granny Smith apple

dried unsulfured cranberries, unsweetened or only sweetened with
apple juice

walnuts instead of pecans (gut repair-friendly when you are farther along)

Preparation

- Preheat oven to 325°F.
- In a large sauté pan, cook bacon over medium heat until done to your
  liking. Some like it crispy and others softer. Drain on paper towel if
  necessary. (If using pork bacon, save leftover fat.)
- In a small bowl, whisk together mustard, optional horseradish, apple
  cider vinegar, and lemon juice and then whisk in oil. Season with pepper.
- Slice Brussels sprouts ⅛–¼ inch (about 30 to 60 cm) thick, using a
  knife or a food processor. You can also pulse them or process into little
  shreds, or use half pulsed and half shredded.
- Transfer veggies to large bowl.
- Preheat large skillet or braiser over medium heat and add 1–2 Tbsp
  coconut or avocado oil (if using pork bacon use leftover fat). Add
  Brussels sprouts and sauté until softened and slightly browned.
- Pour dressing mixture mixture over the sprouts. Then add the balsamic
  vinegar you prefer.
- Add optional pecans (if you are farther along in gut repair), bacon,
  scallions, and optional grapes.
- Place slaw in serving bowl and top with remaining pecans (optional) or
  a few pieces of bacon.
- Serve warm or chilled.

Salmon Salad

This is a delightful protein-rich salad supplement.
Scoop some onto fresh greens any day of the week.
It can be artfully presented to impress guests. They
may think you slaved for hours preparing this,
when it actually took about 30 minutes.

Ingredients

2–3 cans (14 oz/400 g each) wild-caught salmon

2–3 stalks celery, sliced down the middle and chopped

2 cloves garlic, minced

1 (7-oz/200 g) jar of capers (I like to keep the tart salty juice, but drain them if you don't. If you don't have a lime or lemon, the juice can help substitute.)

1-inch/2.5 cm ginger root, peeled and minced

½–1-inch/1.2–2.5 cm turmeric root, peeled and minced

2 Tbsp coconut aminos

2 green onions with green tops, chopped

2 Tbsp freshly chopped dill, or 1 tbsp dried dill

2–3 Tbsp cumin powder, according to taste

¼–½ cup/15–30 g chopped parsley

3 Tbsp olive oil or pea protein base alternative, egg- and soy-free mayonnaise

2 Tbsp olive oil

Juice of one lime or half a lemon, or to taste

sea salt to taste

Options (okay for gut repair)

Olives, sliced

Options (not for gut repair)

½ cup/80 g unsweetened cranberries or currants (you may be able to introduce these earlier; please consult a health care provider)

2 tsp paprika

dash of cayenne

Preparation

- Drain the salmon and flake it into pieces. Combine all ingredients and mix well.
- Pack the salad into a ½-cup measure and mold into a cup shape. Turn the mold over and gently plop on top of any green salad—or fill the trough of a celery stalk—or use as filling for a collard wrap.

- Scoop it up with slices of cucumber. There are so many tasty ways to serve it!

Garnishes
- Make fresh hibiscus flower tea, strain out the flowers, and allow them to cool. Place one or two flowers on top of the salmon cup mold for a beautiful color-contrasting decoration and tasty treat.
- Garnish with green or red grapes after gut repair is complete.

Avocado and Strawberry Salad

This colorful salad is cooling in the summertime and may even get the kids eating greens! This is a transitional recipe, due to the fruit, and is a great way to enjoy a summer salad.

Ingredients

1 medium-large firm but ripe avocado, cut into small cubes or tiny dices

1 cup/160 g sliced fresh organic strawberries

1 tsp ginger root, peeled and minced

½ cup/60 g jicama, peeled and sliced

3–4 Tbsp fresh lime or lemon juice

3 cups/90 g fresh baby spinach leaves, or any salad green, including arugula and sorrel

drizzle of organic olive oil

drizzle of blackberry ginger balsamic or fig balsamic vinegar

sea salt to taste

twist of lemon to taste

Options (very good for gut repair)
sorrel (a slightly sour and highly nutritious light leafy green)

½ cup/60 g Jerusalem artichoke/sunchoke, washed, chopped, diced, or grated. This is a tuber similar to jicama, but slightly less starchy, very crisp, and containing prebiotics to support gut health.

Preparation
- Combine all ingredients except the avocado and salt. Mix well. Gently stir in the avocado dices and dash of salt.
- This dish doesn't keep well. Serve immediately on a bed of baby spinach leaves, mixed spring greens, or arugula with sorrel.

Charly's Raw Kale Salad

Inspired by my friend Charly Wells

This salad is packed with antioxidant and anti-inflammatory power! I was introduced to this at my dear friend Charly's house after a group meditation. Our minds were calm as our bodies became supercharged! **Note:** Due to raw kale's goitrogenic effects (which means it inhibits thyroid function), it is wise to avoid large portions of this salad if you have unresolved thyroid challenges, or do a flash-steam or stir-fry after you've shredded it. I recommend doubling this recipe—you will want leftovers. This makes a pretty salad when garnished with brightly colored grapes.

Ingredients

1 large bunch kale, with stalk/vein removed, and chopped to fit into food processor

1 medium carrot, shredded (approximately ½ cup/25 g shredded carrot)

1 small red or golden beet, shredded (approximately ½ cup/25 g shredded beet)

½ cucumber, cubed

¼ cup/15 g parsley, finely chopped

1 clove garlic, minced

½ inch/1.2 cm fresh ginger root, peeled and diced

juice of ½ lemon, squeezed

3 Tbsp olive oil, or to taste; you can substitute Brazil nut oil for additional selenium, which is great for the thyroid

sea salt to taste

dash of black pepper to taste

dash of balsamic vinegar to taste (try blackberry ginger, black cherry, lavender or fig)

Options (not gut repair-friendly)

¼ cup/40 g dried unsweetened cranberries (might be fine for you during your gut repair, please consult a healthcare provider)

½ cup/50 g organic grapes, sliced in half lengthwise

Preparation

- De-vein and chop kale, and chop the parsley (optional). Pulse the kale and parsley into tiny pieces in a food processor. Add everything to a large bowl and mix well.
- Garnish with red, purple, and/or green grapes (or cranberries after gut repair).

Nopal Salad

Nopal (prickly pear cactus pads) from Mexico, also known as opuntia, is known for its healing properties. It has been shown to help lower blood sugar and HA1c in patients with diabetes. It is also mucilaginous and helps to heal the lining of the stomach and intestines.

Ingredients

4 nopal cactus pads (spines removed)

1 green onion, chopped

1 carrot, shredded

1 clove garlic, diced

2 tsp fresh lime juice or to taste

¼ cup/15 g cilantro, chopped

1 avocado, sliced or cubed

dash of pink sea salt and pepper to taste

Options (gut repair-friendly)

1 Tbsp fresh ginger, peeled and grated

2 Tbsp basil chiffonade

Options (not gut repair-friendly for the first 2–4 months)

1 large tomato, chopped

Preparation

- Chop nopal cactus pads into small squares, place in a saucepan, and boil for 15–20 minutes, then drain.
- Chop the green onion, garlic, and cilantro; shred the carrot; and squeeze lime juice, and combine in a large bowl. Add boiled nopal cactus, and gently mix.
- Serve with avocado on top and a drizzle of olive oil. **Note:** You can also serve on a bed of fresh spinach.

Caramelized Fennel Salad

Ingredients

2 large fennel bulbs

½ orange, zested

5–10 fresh mint leaves (to taste, but approx. 2 heaping Tbsp)

2 Tbsp Dijon mustard

¼ cup/60 ml olive oil

3 Tbsp ghee or avocado oil or coconut oil for cooking

1 clove garlic, crushed (optional)

sea salt and pepper to taste

Preparation

- In a small bowl whisk together a light dressing of olive oil, Dijon mustard, orange zest, optional crushed garlic, salt and pepper to taste. Set aside.
- Chop fennel bulb into 1-inch or 2.5 cm pieces. Save the fennel tops for bone broth or chicken stock.
- In a large skillet with a tight-fitting lid, heat cooking oil over medium-high. Add fennel, and season with coarse salt and ground pepper. Cook, stirring occasionally, until mixture begins to brown, about 5 minutes. Reduce heat to medium, cover, and cook 5–7 minutes. Uncover, add 1 Tbsp water, and cook, stirring constantly, until golden brown and soft, 2 minutes. Remove from stove.
- While fennel is cooking, chiffonade the mint leaves, if they are too tiny, then just add them whole. Place fennel in a serving bowl, drizzle with the dressing, and top with fresh mint leaves.
- Serve warm with a protein or atop a bed of fresh or lightly steamed greens.

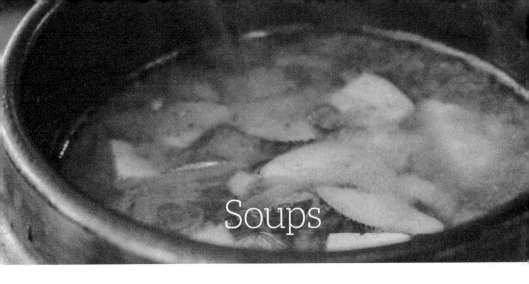

Soups

Chicken Soup for the Soul . . . and the Gut

This soup is a staple in our gut-healing household. I borrowed the idea from the GAPS diet minus the gut-damaging whey and eggs allowed by GAPS. (GAPS stands for "Gut and Psychology Syndrome") It is easy to heat for any meal, take in a thermos to work, serve to last-minute guests, or bring to an ill friend. When doing intensive gut repair, I encourage people to make a huge batch, store it in the fridge and/or freezer, and eat it for at least two meals per day, in a rotating nutritional plan. It helps decrease inflammation, alleviates bloating, restores energy, and is satisfyingly filling. Please check the options below for more ideas. It's not what Grandma used to make—it's better!

Ingredients

2–3 lbs/1–1.5 kg boneless skinless chicken meat (I prefer thighs— more flavor and fat)

1 large fennel bulb, chopped into 1-inch or smaller pieces (use only the white bulb, save the green stalks for homemade broth)

3–4 carrots, quartered lengthwise and sliced thin

1 large parsnip, quartered lengthwise and sliced thin

1 onion, chopped

3–4 stalks celery, cut down the middle and chopped

1 cup/150 g broccoli florets, more if you love them or less if you are sensitive to cruciferous veggies and they cause a lot of gas and bloating—incorporate them gradually as your gut repairs, or consider adding digestive enzymes and HCl to your regimen. Consult your holistic healthcare provider

1 cup/150 g cauliflower florets

1 large zucchini/courgette, chopped

1 small or half of a large butternut squash, not peeled, but seeded and chopped

1 large yellow summer squash, chopped

½ cup/30 g parsley, chopped

2 large garlic cloves

1–2 inches/2.5–5 cm of ginger root, peeled and chopped

1–2 inches/2.5–5 cm of turmeric root, peeled and chopped

2–3 Tbsp rosemary, dried

2–3 Tbsp thyme, dried

1 Tbsp oregano, dried

4–8 cups/1–2 l chicken stock, homemade is best

sea salt and pepper to taste

Optional (okay for gut repair)

1–2 cups/150 g Brussels sprouts (if you have gas, GI pain, or abdominal bloating, don't use these)

1 cup/90 g purple or green cabbage (same warning as above)

8–10 stalks asparagus ends, trimmed and then chopped into 1-inch or 2.5 cm pieces (avoid with gout symptoms)

2 stalks collard greens (I trim the bottom stalk off and leave the rest)

2 stalks kale (I trim the bottom stalk off and leave the rest)

Preparation

- Cook chicken and stock in a large pot on medium-high heat.
- While chicken is cooking, begin chopping vegetables. I separate the firmer veggies from the softer ones. Broccoli, carrots, parsnip, ginger, turmeric, garlic, fennel bulb, butternut squash, and optional Brussels sprouts are firmer. Zucchini, yellow squash, celery, parsley, and cabbage (optional) are softer and cook faster. Certain veggies can be shredded with the food processor attachment—carrots, parsnips, zucchini, yellow squash, Brussels sprouts, fennel—the rest require chopping.
- When chicken is fully cooked, remove with a slotted spoon and add to the food processor. Pulse a few times until it is shredded. Return to the pot.
- Add firmer veggies to the shredded chicken and stock. Reduce heat to medium and cook covered for 10 minutes.
- Add softer veggies except the parsley, and cook covered on low for 5 minutes. Turn off heat, and allow veggies to sit covered in the hot pot for 15 minutes. They will continue to cook.
- Add parsley at the end and serve immediately, or store for future meals. Garnish with avocado slices and a drizzle of olive oil.

Creamy Spiced Cauliflower Soup

Ingredients

1 medium head cauliflower (about 2 lbs/1 kg), trimmed and broken into florets

2 celery stalks, chopped

1 small leek, chopped (about 2 cups/200 g)

4 cups/1 l vegetable or chicken broth

1 Tbsp cumin seeds

1 Tbsp coriander seeds

2 tsp fennel seeds

1 Tbsp avocado oil as needed

2 cloves garlic, minced

2 tsp minced fresh ginger root or 1 tsp powdered ginger

1 tsp sea salt and pepper to taste

2 Tbsp freshly chopped chives or cilantro

½ lime, juice used at the end

1 cup/240 ml full-fat coconut milk (optional for a higher-fat-content soup)

Optional (not gut repair-friendly; use after 2–4 months of gut repair)

¼ cup/25 g toasted sliced almonds

pinch of cayenne

Preparation

- Combine cumin, coriander, and fennel seeds in a small skillet over medium heat. Toast, shaking the pan frequently, until fragrant and spices begin to darken (about 3 minutes). Let cool. Grind to a powder with a mortar and pestle or spice grinder.
- Heat oil in a large saucepan or soup pot over medium heat. Add leeks and cook, stirring frequently, until they begin to soften, 4–6 minutes. Add the ground spices, garlic, ginger, salt, and cayenne. Stir to combine. Stir in cauliflower, and cook, stirring, for 2–3 minutes. Add broth, and bring to a gentle simmer. Partially cover, reduce heat to maintain a gentle simmer and cook until the cauliflower is tender, about 25 minutes.
- Use a slotted spoon to remove about 1 cup/150 g of the cauliflower. Let cool slightly. Chop into small florets.
- Working in batches, purée the rest of the soup in a blender, and return it to the pot or purée in the pot with an immersion blender. (Use caution when puréeing hot liquids.) Add a squeeze of lime juice to taste. Serve garnished with the reserved florets, almonds (after gut repair), and chives (or cilantro).

Tip: For the best flavor, toast chopped nuts or seeds. Heat a dry skillet over medium-low heat. Add nuts or seeds and cook, stirring constantly, until fragrant, 2–4 minutes.

Sweet Potato Cranberry Soup

This soup is beautiful! The colorful addition of cranberries makes it a simple and stunning dish to serve with any main course. It can be prepared in advance and refrigerated for 2 days, or frozen for 1 month. Serve it hot, topped with a drizzle of cranberry purée. This is a transitional recipe. It is higher in carbohydrate than most soups, so be mindful of how your body may react. If you're restricting carbohydrates until later in your gut-repair program, save it for a special treat—it'll be worth the wait! If you are ketogenic, then limit consumption to ¾ cup/180 ml.

Soup Ingredients

1 large onion, coarsely chopped

4 carrots, coarsely chopped

3 lbs/1.5 kg sweet potatoes, cubed (smaller cubes cook faster)

2–3 Tbsp coconut oil

2–3 Tbsp coconut butter

1 can or jar (12–16 oz/180–240 ml) prepared whole cranberry sauce, no sugar added, best if homemade

4–5 cups/1–1.25 l gluten-free, dairy-free vegetable or chicken broth—homemade is best!

1 tsp ground ginger, or a smidgeon more, to taste

1 tsp ground cinnamon, or a smidgeon more, to taste

1 tsp pink or gray salt, or to taste

½ tsp white or tri-colored pepper

parsley, to garnish

Secret Cranberry Sauce Ingredients

1 bag (10 oz/280 g) whole cranberries, fresh or frozen

1 cup/240 ml water or fresh-squeezed orange juice

Note: The orange juice could impact your ketosis, so listen to your body. It is also high in sugar, so wait 2 months before you use it. It depends on how strict you are being. Use water instead.

1 tsp orange zest

stevia or monk fruit, a few drops to taste (don't over-sweeten—it should be tart, as a counterpoint to the sweet soup)

Option (okay for gut repair)

1 Tbsp coconut butter

Option (not for gut repair)

¾ **tsp ground nutmeg** (may be fine depending on your gut; please consult your healthcare provider)

Preparation

- Preheat oven to 400°F.
- Toss onions, carrots, and sweet potatoes in coconut oil and roast them in a large heavy roasting pan for 45 minutes, stirring every 10–15 minutes.
- While the vegetables are cooking, purée cranberry sauce ingredients in a blender until smooth. Set aside.
- Place roasted vegetables in a large stockpot. Add broth, optional nutmeg, ginger, cinnamon, salt, and pepper. Cover, and simmer for 15 minutes or until the vegetables are very soft.
- In a heavy-duty blender or food processor, purée the hot soup in batches. Add broth as needed to achieve desired consistency.
  Note: Take extra care when processing hot liquids in a blender! Hot soup will expand when processed, so don't fill the blender more than half full. To avoid being burned by soup spatter, drape a dishtowel over the covered blender.
- Ladle hot soup into individual bowls, and drizzle cranberry purée decoratively over the top of each serving. I use a cake frosting decorating bag to squeeze out cranberry sauce on top of the soup. Garnish with a bit of parsley.

Butternut Bisque

This beautifully orange bisque really hits the spot in autumn. If you're ketogenic or limiting carbohydrate intake, just have ½–¾ cup for now. It is worth it! This is more of a transitional recipe unless eaten in small amounts and in the evening. This is one of my in-laws' favorite recipes. Chuck has an aversion to vegetables, but this soup hit the spot for him, and I bet it will for you, too!

Ingredients

1 medium or 2 small butternut squashes, washed well, not peeled, seeded and cubed

1 medium yellow onion, chopped

2–4 cups/500 ml–1 l chicken or veggie broth

1–2 cans/380–760 ml coconut milk

1–2 inches/2.5–5 cm fresh ginger root, peeled and minced

sea salt and pepper to taste

⅓ cup/20 g parsley, chopped for garnish

Option (gut-repair friendliness depends on your diet plan)

1–2 large apples (Fuji, Gala, or Granny Smith are best)

Preparation

- Cook squash, onion, and ginger in broth. The squash should be mostly, but not completely, submerged in broth. Cook until squash is almost tender. (Possibly add apple, according to your gut and blood sugar health. Cook another 5 minutes.)
- Purée in batches in a heavy-duty blender or food processor. Return purée to soup pot, add the can of coconut milk, salt and pepper, then heat on high for 2 minutes, stirring frequently.
- Serve garnished with freshly chopped parsley.

Homemade Chicken Bone Broth

Preparing your own chicken bone broth makes good economic and nutritional sense. Rather than buy broth, make your own, get the chicken meat for free, and get money back to cover the cost of the broth's vegetables and the gas or electricity needed to cook it overnight!

There are two schools of thought regarding the easiest approach to making bone broth. My husband prefers to make a large double batch less often. We used to have a second refrigerator in our garage, so we could easily store as many as 10 quart bottles. Our friend Annette makes broth one chicken at a time. She has only one refrigerator, so 10 quarts is far too much. She slow-cooks the chicken in an electric crock, then strips the carcass of meat, adds water and vegetables, and cooks the broth right in the crock. No stock pot is necessary, and there's just one clean-up job for the chicken dinner and the broth making. She stores broth in the freezer in 8-oz /240 ml jelly jars, which are very convenient for a single meal.

Ingredients

1 carcass from a 5–6-lb chicken
(or two carcasses of 3-lb)

5 quarts/5 l water

2 carrots, diced or shredded

2 stalks celery, diced or shredded

1 onion, diced or shredded

1 small bunch parsley, chopped

2 clove garlic, pressed or minced

¼ cup/60 m apple cider vinegar

2 chicken feet (optional)—I found
them at my CSA from a local
organic farmer

1 tsp sea salt

Few dashes of pepper

1 tsp rosemary, thyme, oregano,
basil (optional)

Any other bones from beef or
ox are welcome, or you can
do a different beef bone broth;
simply substitute the chicken
carcass for beef, buffalo, or ox
bones.

Miscellaneous vegetable scraps
you might have saved—I save
fennel stalks, broccoli stalks,
zucchini ends, you name it . . .

Preparation

- Prepare all vegetables. I use a food processor shredder attachment.
  Combine all ingredients in stockpot or crockpot. Bring to a boil, then
  simmer for 8–24 hours.
- Strain out all solid matter, pour liquid into glass jars or bottles and keep
  refrigerated, or freeze. Use for making soups, and add to concentrated
  soups to increase liquid content.

Creamy Parsnip Andouille Soup

Sausage makes this creamy soup hearty, yet it has a light
finish. If you are on a strict ketogenic diet, do your best to consume
½–¾ cup/120–180 ml at a time, preferably in the evening. This can
be used as a transitional recipe. It is scrumptious, and you will be
tempted to have more, but the parsnips create higher starch content.
Feel free to add more collards and kale—it's up to your palate.

Ingredients

1½–2 lbs/750 g–1 kg parsnips,
chopped (smaller ones are less
fibrous)

1 large onion, chopped

2–3 stalks celery, chopped

2 cloves garlic, sliced

12–24 oz/340–680 g Andouille
sausage—turkey, buffalo, or
chicken

2 medium leaves of collard
  greens, de-stemmed/
  de-veined and chopped
2 large leaves of kale,
  de-stemmed/de-veined and
  chopped

1–2 Tbsp dried rosemary
6–8 cups/1–2 l chicken or turkey
  broth
3 Tbsp coconut or avocado oil
sea salt and black pepper to
  taste

Preparation

- Sauté onion and garlic in oil until the onions become translucent. Add parsnips and celery. Stir-fry for 5 minutes.
- If the sausages are raw, begin by cooking them in a frying pan. Chop cooked sausages into bite-sized pieces. If the sausages are thick, you might need to slice them lengthwise before chopping.
- Add stir-fried sausage and veggies, rosemary, and broth to a soup pot, and bring to a boil. Cook another 5 minutes, or until parsnips are tender. If your soup pot is heavy, you can sauté and stir-fry in it directly and have one less pan to clean.
- Purée in batches in a heavy-duty blender or food processor. Return to the soup pot, and add sausage. Lower heat to medium-low.
- Add chopped collards and kale. Add salt and pepper. Cook another 5 minutes, until the collards and kale begin to look bright green.

Russian Borscht

This vibrantly deep red soup will nourish you throughout the winter and spring seasons. It's filled with a beautiful array of veggies, representing all Five Elements and all flavors of Traditional Chinese Medicine. Notice how many of the vegetables affect the liver and support the spleen and pancreas. A great transitional recipe, or even ketogenic if eaten in small amounts (½–¾ cup /120–180 ml in the evening), this soup helps harmonize the dynamic and delicate balance among the Five Elements.

Ingredients

1 cup/130 g parsnips, chopped
1–2 cups/130–260 g beets, chopped
1½ cups/220 g onion, chopped

4 cups/1 l stock or water (I use
  homemade chicken bone
  broth, see recipe in this book)

2 Tbsp olive oil

1 Tbsp caraway seeds

2 tsp sea salt

2 stalks celery, chopped

2–3 large carrots, sliced

2 cups/180 g purple cabbage, sliced

¼ cup/15 g parsley, chopped

2 Tbsp fresh dill, minced, or to taste (I often use more because I love it!)

1 Tbsp apple cider vinegar or coconut vinegar

black pepper to taste

Options (not for gut repair)
1 cup/240 g tomatoes, puréed or diced
Garnish with fresh chopped tomato

Preparation

- Place parsnips, beets, and water or stock in a saucepan. and cook until almost tender. Save the liquid.
- In a large kettle or soup pot, begin frying the onions in olive oil. Add caraway seeds and salt. Fry until the onions are translucent.
- Add celery, carrots, and cabbage. Add saved liquid, and cook covered until all vegetables are almost tender.
- Add beets, parsnips, and all remaining ingredients. Cover, and simmer slowly for about 30 minutes. Taste, and adjust seasoning as you like.
- Serve topped with extra dill or garnish with a little parsley.

Kristin's Kimchi Soup

This Korean fermented soup is excellent for gut repair! Fermentation is an ancient process whereby carbohydrates are broken down by microorganisms. The byproducts of this process are actually good for us and are both prebiotic and probiotic, supporting healthy intestinal flora. Fermented foods have been shown to aid in digestion, increase digestive enzymes, enhance immune function, help us fend off harmful bacteria, and even fight cancer. They can also chelate—draw out—harmful toxins such as heavy metals.

Omit the horseradish if you don't like it spicy. The burdock root is bitter, and if you're not used to it, you may wish to start small, but it's excellent for liver detoxification. You'll need a large ceramic bowl and a smaller heavy cover that will press the veggies down and keep them submerged at all times. I use a Le Creuset 6-quart bowl and a saucepan lid to submerge the veggies. **Note:** If you are sensitive to histamine, then it's best to avoid fermented foods.

I've listed my favorite veggies, but you may choose any root veggies you prefer. This recipe makes a big batch, which I like to refrigerate and eat over a period of several weeks. You might wish to start smaller.

Ingredients

4 liters filtered water (do not use plain tap water, since chlorine can inhibit fermentation)

½ cup/25 g dulse (seaweed). Omit if you have Hashimoto's thyroiditis or other thyroid challenges; in some people, iodine-containing foods can worsen the condition while others can benefit

1 burdock root, well-scrubbed and chopped into rounds

1 turnip, cubed or cut into julienne strips

1–2 parsnips, chopped into rounds or julienne strips

1 daikon radish, chopped

1 small red or yellow beet, chopped

2–3 inches/5–7.5 cm ginger root, peeled and grated or chopped

2 inches/5 cm horseradish (more if you like it hot), peeled and chopped

1–2 cups/90–180 g cabbage (purple, green, or Napa), chopped into bite-sized chunks

2–3 cloves garlic, sliced or cut into chunks

1 small yellow onion, chopped

2 carrots, cut into rounds or long julienne strips

½–¾ cup/150–225 g ground sea salt

Preparation

- Combine all ingredients in a large bowl. Add salt gradually—it should taste salty, but not repulsively so.
- Place small lid in bowl so that it presses the veggies down into the water. Don't allow veggies to sneak above the lid; they must remain submerged. Some liquid will rise above the lid.
- Set the bowl aside at room temperature. *Do not refrigerate.*
- Stir twice a day, once in the morning and again in the evening. Be careful to replace the lid so that all veggies are submerged.
- During the warmer summer months, kimchi takes 5–7 days to ferment. If your summers are hot, it might take only 4 days. It will get a little bubbly, which is a sign of healthy fermentation. Taste periodically to

gauge progress. The veggies will soften over time. If, by the second day, it no longer tastes salty, then add a little more, one tablespoon at a time. There's an art to it. Trust that you'll find your way!

- When fermentation is complete, you're ready to bottle. I use mason jars with sealed lids. Ladle the veggies and juice into jars, cover, and refrigerate. If you have brine—the salty liquid—left over, place it in a jar and save it in the fridge for use as a starter for your next batch, which will make it ferment more quickly.
- Eat as you please for breakfast, lunch, dinner, or as a snack. It makes great road food or a camping treat!

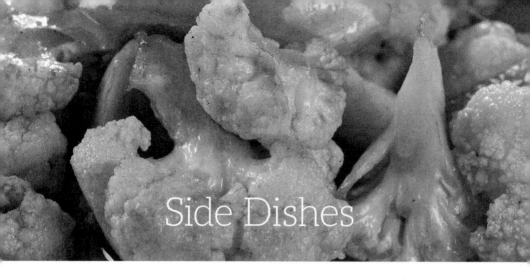

Side Dishes

Cauliflower Rice

This is my husband's favorite rice substitute, and it works
like a charm. I've had guests ask, "What kind of rice is
this? It's so delicious!" They never guess it's a vegetable!
It's excellent with any dish that benefits from something
soaking up delicious juices; all of my children have been
fooled by it, even the pickiest of them. Also great on its own.

Ingredients

1 cauliflower head

3 Tbsp coconut oil (I prefer refined
for this recipe—I like to cook with
coconut and drizzle afterward with
olive oil), **or use ghee, grapeseed,
avocado oil, or duck fat**

1–2 cloves garlic, minced

2 Tbsp flat-leaf parsley, chopped

½ tsp sea salt, or to taste

Cracked black pepper to taste

Options

Sauté an **onion** with the oil and then add the garlic.
Sauté **½–1 cup/50–100 g chopped celery** in oil before adding the cauliflower.
Pinch of saffron

Variation

Add basil instead of parsley to combine with dishes that benefit from
basil, such as certain Thai curry dishes. If you use basil, to avoid bruising
and maintain the flavor, try the chiffonade technique and stack the
individual leaves, roll them up into a cigar shape, and cut across the roll to
create long streamers of basil.

Preparation

- Cut the cauliflower into florets, and place in steamer. When soft enough to pierce with a fork, cool slightly, and add to food processor. Pulse the steamed cauliflower until it is the texture of rice. You may have to do this in a couple of batches. Or smash with a potato masher or dice with a knife.
- Place the cauliflower in a medium bowl and set aside.
- Heat the oil in a large skillet over medium-high heat. Add the garlic, and sauté for about 30 seconds, being careful not to burn the garlic. **Note:** For a stronger garlic taste and more medicinal use, add the garlic after the cauliflower has cooked a bit.
- Add the cauliflower to the pan, and stir-fry for 5–10 minutes, until tender.
- Add the parsley and the sea salt (and optional cracked black pepper) to taste.

You may add various other sauces to the rice, and serve with chicken, Moroccan lamb, and Indian dishes. The sky is the limit! Serves 4–6.

Indian Creamy Spinach Malai Sak

This is another of my husband's favorites! This dish combines authentic Indian flavors with gut repair-friendly ingredients. If you have an aversion to cooked spinach, this may convert you to loving it!

Ingredients

⅛ tsp cayenne pepper (see options below)
½ tsp ground coriander
¼ tsp ground pepper
⅛ tsp ground nutmeg (see options below)
½ tsp turmeric
1–2 tsp Garam Masala to taste
3 Tbsp water

4 Tbsp coconut oil or ghee (lactose- and casein-free)
1 lb/500 g fresh spinach, trimmed and washed (chop it up if using large-leaf rather than baby spinach)
½ cup/120 ml original, unsweetened coconut kefir (check ingredients!)

Options

For very strict gut repair, omit cayenne and nutmeg; however, the nutmeg is really a special flavor here, so just this once, I give you full permission to incorporate it, as long as you check with your healthcare provider first!

Preparation

- Combine spices in a small bowl, add the water, and mix well.
- Melt the coconut oil in a large quart or liter pan with a lid. Add the spice and water mixture to the oil and then pack in the spinach, and sprinkle with salt.
- Cover, and reduce the heat. Cook for about 5 minutes, then turn the leaves over, and cook for a few more minutes.
- Remove from the heat, add the coconut kefir, and stir well. If you don't have coconut kefir, canned full-fat coconut milk is a great substitute.
- Serve immediately and enjoy!

Caribbean-Inspired Carrots

Bugs Bunny would do backflips for this dish! It has a higher sugar content, due to the carrots, so if you're aiming for ketogenic, only have ½–¾ cup/100–150 g or less per serving, and in the evening. This is a great transitional recipe.

Ingredients

2 Tbsp coconut oil, ghee, or avocado oil

1½ cup/225 g yellow onion, minced

1 heaping Tbsp fresh ginger root, peeled and minced

2 tsp garlic, minced

½ tsp sea salt or to taste

2 lbs/1 kg carrots, cut on the diagonal into ¼-inch-thick slices

2 Tbsp fresh lemon or lime juice

½ cup/40 g shredded unsweetened coconut

Option (okay for gut repair)

Add 2–4 Tbsp of coconut butter, before adding the shredded coconut.

Preparation

- Preheat oven to 375°F. Coat the bottom of a glass or Pyrex baking dish, and set aside.

- Place a large, deep skillet over medium heat. Allow it to heat for about a minute, then add the remaining oil to coat pan. Add the onion and ginger, and sauté for 5 minutes. Stir in the garlic and half the salt, and sauté for another 5 minutes.
- Add the carrots and the remaining salt, and stir until the carrots are well coated with the onion mixture. Turn down the heat, and cover. Cook for another 5 minutes undisturbed.
- Add the lemon or lime juice, and cook covered for another 5 minutes.
- Transfer everything to the baking dish, and cover with a lid (or foil).
- Bake for 20 minutes, or until the carrots are fork-tender. Uncover, sprinkle with shredded coconut, and return to the oven uncovered until the coconut is golden, about 5–10 minutes longer.
- Serve warm.

Whipped Clouds of Flavor

This is a substitute for mashed potatoes. The flavors can vary, depending on which root vegetables you choose. It won't taste like regular mashed potatoes but will appear similar. The flavor is much more sophisticated and nutrient-dense. This is an excellent transitional recipe, but due to the root vegetables it has a slightly higher starch content, so ketogenic folks, eat it sparingly—about ½ cup /100 g or less.

Ingredients

1 small-medium celery root, scrubbed and cubed (no need to peel)

1 medium-large parsnip, chopped

1 small-medium rutabaga, chopped

1 burdock root, peeled and chopped

1 small-medium turnip, chopped

1 medium yellow beet, chopped

4 Tbsp coconut oil, or ghee, as needed for consistency

2–3 Tbsp coconut butter (optional)

½ cup/120 ml coconut kefir (optional)

sea salt and pepper to taste

½ cup/30 g parsley, chopped, for garnish

chicken broth, as needed for consistency

Option (okay for gut repair)
Add chopped **fennel bulb** to the mix

Preparation

- Scrub and chop all root veggies. Place in a pan, and steam until fork-tender.
- Transfer all ingredients, including oil, to a food processor or blender, and blend until smooth (you may need to do this in batches to avoid overfilling processor/blender with hot mixture).
- Garnish with chopped parsley (optional).

Herbes de Provence Roasted Vegetables

These roasted vegetables perfectly accompany almost any simple meat dish, such as Crockpot Chicken. The Herbes de Provence herb mixture (which you can find in most any grocery store) adds a lovely flavor. These herbs may come whole, so you may choose to grind them into a powder or leave larger pieces of herbs on the veggies. Both will work fine. Feel free to include other veggies or omit any listed below that you don't care for (just keep it within the gut-repair program). You can chop everything small and add to a roasting pan, or keep the vegetables in longer pieces. Make sure to cut them thinly enough so that they roast through. **Note:** The more root veggies you use, the more transitional this recipe is. If you wish to remain ketogenic then avoid large amounts of sweet potatoes or winter squash in this recipe.

These make wonderful leftovers and can be easily reheated in a toaster oven (not a microwave!) at work for lunch the following day.

Ingredients

2 large leeks, chopped lengthwise in half

2–3 large carrots, halved lengthwise and cut in half

1–2 zucchini/courgette, cut into ½-inch rounds

1 small sweet potato, cut into ¼-inch-thick rounds, then cut rounds in half

1 large fennel bulb or two smaller ones, stems removed, and cut into thin rounds or pieces

asparagus, as many stalks as you please

broccoli florets and stalk, cut lengthwise and quartered

cauliflower florets and stalk, cut lengthwise and quartered

3 cloves garlic, sliced

1 turnip, cut into ¼-inch thick rounds and then cut rounds in half

1 sweet onion, sliced, optional

½ butternut squash, cut into ¼–½ inch rounds and then quartered

1 cup/150 g Brussels sprouts, halved, or as many as you please

salt and pepper

2–3 tsp Herbes de Provence or to taste

4 Tbsp coconut or avocado oil or ghee (lactose- and casein-free)

Option (okay for gut repair if it contains no yeast or other contaminants)

1 bouillon cube can be crushed and sprinkled over vegetables

Preparation

- Preheat oven to 400°F. Arrange veggies in a roasting pan. Brush with coconut, ghee, or avocado oil, and season with salt, pepper, and Herbes de Provence.
- Roast in oven until you can easily pierce the winter squash and sweet potato, about 50 minutes. Flip the vegetables over halfway through cooking, sprinkle with more salt, pepper, and Herbes de Provence, and brush or drizzle with more oil if necessary.
- Remove from oven, allow to cool for 5 minutes and then serve.

Keto Roasted Turmeric Cauliflower

Ingredients

1 head of cauliflower

1 Tbsp coconut oil, avocado oil, ghee, or grapeseed oil

1 Tbsp turmeric

pinch of cumin

salt and pepper to taste

olive oil for drizzling when serving

Option (not gut repair-friendly)

Add **½ cup/60 g roasted hazelnuts** (after 2 months of gut repair has been completed).

Preparation

- Preheat oven to 400° F. Chop cauliflower head into florets, and transfer to a baking dish. Add oil, turmeric, cumin, and salt, and mix.
- Cover baking dish with foil to keep florets from drying out, and roast for 35–40 minutes.
- Remove foil, and cook for another 15 minutes; you could also broil them for 5 minutes until golden.

Carrot Timbales

This gorgeous side dish can accompany almost any main dish. It has a mild flavor and lovely presentation. Ketogenic folks should only consume ½–¾ cup/100–150 g in the evening, and not daily. One cup of cooked carrots has approximately 12.3 grams of carbohydrates.

Ingredients

2 Tbsp coconut oil or ghee (lactose- and casein-free)

1 lb/450 g carrots, washed and cut in half lengthwise, then sliced

1 clove garlic, minced

¼ tsp sea salt or to taste

1 tsp fresh thyme, minced or dried

⅛ cup/30 ml coconut milk

2 Tbsp chia seeds, ground

2 tsp Italian parsley, chopped, to garnish

Option (okay for gut repair)

1 tsp ginger powder, or 1–2 tsp curry powder and turmeric (either powdered or fresh root, peeled and minced)

Options (not for gut repair, but excellent flavor enhancers!)

½ tsp sweet paprika

1 pinch nutmeg

Preparation

- Heat oil in a heavy saucepan. When hot, add carrots and garlic, and toss to coat with oil. Cook covered over medium-low heat until tender, about 30 minutes.
- Preheat oven to 350°F. Lightly grease six ½-cup/120 ml ramekins. Set aside.
- Transfer cooked carrot mixture into food processor. Add salt (optional paprika and nutmeg), thyme, and coconut milk, and purée until

smooth. Add ground chia seeds, and purée for about 1 minute, until well combined.

- Spoon carrot purée into ramekins, and fill almost to the top.
- Place timbales on a cookie sheet, and bake in the oven for 40–45 minutes.
- Either serve in ramekins, or unmold by running a knife around sides of the ramekins.
- Serve warm or slightly chilled, garnished with chopped parsley.

Raw Stuffing

Thanksgiving dinner in the United States wouldn't be the same without stuffing. You needn't be deprived any longer! No breadcrumbs—just veggies and herbs—which means no bloating or further gut damage. Enjoy leaving the table without having to extend your belt buckle.

Ingredients

2 cups/200 g celery, cut into ¼-inch slices
1½ cups/180 g zucchini/ courgette, small cubes
¼ cup/60 g thinly sliced leek
1 Tbsp fresh rosemary, minced

2 tsp fresh thyme, minced
1 tsp rubbed sage
1 Tbsp olive oil
¼ tsp sea salt
1 tsp coconut aminos

Option (okay for gut repair)
1 Tbsp basil chiffonade

Options (not for gut repair)
¼ cup/40 g dried, unsweetened cranberries (this may be okay for you during gut repair; consult your healthcare professional)
½ cup/65 g sunflower seeds, pine nuts, or pecans (generally safe for this one special meal)
¼ cup/40 g raisins (too sweet for strict gut repair)

Preparation
- Place all of the ingredients, except the raisins or cranberries, in a mixing bowl, and stir well to coat evenly with the oil and spices.

- If you have a dehydrator, set it to 145°F, and heat the food for about an hour, stirring occasionally to keep the top hydrated. You can use your oven if it's possible to set the temperature to 145°F.
- If using raisins or cranberries, add after dehydrating, and stir well.
- Serve immediately, or store in an airtight container for up to 4 days.

Creamed Spinach

This spinach dish can convert just about anyone into loving cooked spinach. You may not have thought to combine spinach and coconut, but they complement each other quite nicely. At first glance, the blanching may seem like a "job," but it does go fast and is worth the small amount of effort.

Ingredients

1 lb/500 g baby spinach
½ cup/120 ml coconut milk
3 cloves garlic, minced
½ tsp coconut flour

2 tsp coconut oil or ghee
(lactose- and casein-free)
1 shallot, minced
sea salt and pepper to taste

Option (okay for gut repair)
¼ cup/60 ml coconut kefir (add at the end, as cooking kills the probiotics)

Option (not for gut repair, but it's just a bit)
½ tsp paprika

Option (not for gut repair)
Garnish with pine nuts

Preparation

- Boil a pot of water large enough to hold the spinach and blanch it. Submerge spinach for 30 seconds, or until bright green.
- Remove spinach using a slotted spoon, or dump into colander, and drain. Immediately transfer spinach to bowl of ice water. Drain, squeeze out all the moisture, and roughly chop larger leaves; it may be unnecessary to chop the baby leaves.

- Heat the coconut milk in a small saucepan over medium heat. Add 2 tsp of minced garlic (helps to infuse the coconut milk with the garlic flavor).
- Whisk in the ½ tsp coconut flour until slightly simmering. Remove from heat.
- Meanwhile, heat coconut oil or ghee in a skillet over medium heat, and add shallot, remaining garlic, and optional paprika. Cook until shallots are just translucent (be careful not to burn the shallots or garlic).
- Add the spinach and coconut cream sauce, and simmer until everything is cooked through. Then add the optional coconut kefir.
- Serve immediately.

Bitter Greens with a Sweet and Sour Surprise

I don't often combine fruits with vegetables, but this is one exception that I had to share with you! This is a transitional recipe that is detoxifying and nourishing for the liver, kidneys, and blood. The bitter flavors assist in digestion and enhance cardiovascular health. Don't pull and trash those dandelion weeds! Use them in this recipe! Avoid picking dandelion growing along roadsides or in dog parks to avoid contamination.

Ingredients

2 Tbsp coconut or avocado oil, or ghee (lactose- and casein-free)
1–2 cups/150–300 g sweet onions (try sweet Vidalias), sliced
3 large bunches of fresh greens, stemmed and coarsely chopped (about 12 cups). I use beet greens, mustard greens, collards, dandelion, and kale in any combination.
1 cup/160 g fresh pitted sour cherries or unsweetened canned cherries, drained, or dried cherries
sea salt and ground black pepper to taste

Options (okay for gut repair)

twist of lemon for garnish
1 Tbsp coconut aminos or to taste

Preparation

- Coat a large, deep skillet with oil, and set over medium heat. Sauté the onions for about 5 minutes. Cover and allow to cook until very tender.
- Add the greens in batches. Sprinkle salt between the layer of greens. Turn the greens with tongs or spatula, moving the wilted ones from the bottom to the top.
- When all the greens are a vibrant green color and a bit wilted, stir in the cherries, and cook for about 2 more minutes.
- Serve on a platter with a sprinkle of black pepper, an optional twist of lemon, or a dash of coconut aminos

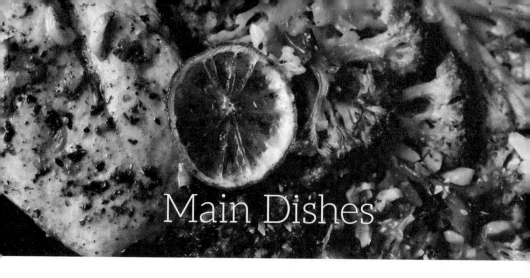

Main Dishes

Chicken Alfredo with Broccoli

Ingredients

4 chicken breasts, baked, either whole or cubed meat

4 cups/500 g broccoli florets, loosely measured, about 10 oz/280 g

4 cups/500 g zucchini/ courgette, sliced

½ tbsp grapeseed or avocado oil

½ tbsp Italian seasoning

Optional (not gut repair-friendly; use after 2–4 months of gut repair)
1 cup/75 g mushrooms, chopped

Alfredo Sauce

4 cloves garlic, minced or pressed

1 Tbsp olive oil

1 cup/240 ml unsweetened coconut milk (or after 2–4 months of gut repair, use almond or Brazil nut milk)

½ cup/120 ml vegetable broth

¼ cup/60 ml lemon juice, less for less dominant lemon flavor

1 head cauliflower, chopped into florets, about 2 heaping cups

salt and pepper to taste

Preparation

- Preheat oven to 450°F, and line a large, rimmed baking sheet with a silicone mat.
- On the baking sheet, combine broccoli, ½ Tbsp olive oil, Italian seasoning, and a pinch of salt, and toss to combine. Spread the broccoli and zucchini in a single layer.
- Roast broccoli and zucchini for 15 minutes, stirring halfway through, or until broccoli and zucchini is crisp-tender and beginning to lightly brown.

- Remove from oven, and set aside.
- **Note:** If using mushrooms, stir-fry now, and add at the end.

Alfredo Sauce

- Heat a large sauté pan over medium heat. Once hot, add 1 Tbsp olive oil and garlic, and sauté for 30 seconds.
- Slowly whisk in coconut milk, vegetable broth, and lemon juice, and bring it to a simmer.
- Add chopped cauliflower, and season with salt and pepper. Simmer for 7–10 minutes, or until the cauliflower is soft.
- Remove from the heat, and carefully pour the mixture into a blender. Process on high setting until smooth. Season with salt and pepper.
- Pour sauce over broccoli, zucchini, and chicken, and serve warm.

Note: The sauce does dry out as time goes by, which is why I make extra sauce for this recipe. Add more sauce as you see fit!

Wild Salmon with Lemon Dill Sauce

This simple salmon dish can be served throughout the year but is best during fresh salmon season. Remember to purchase wild salmon and avoid farmed.

Ingredients

1½ lbs/750 g wild salmon (sockeye, or whatever is in season)

1 Tbsp lemon zest

2 Tbsp coconut or avocado oil, or ghee

1–2 Tbsp or more fresh or dried dill, chopped, for garnish

1 lemon, for juice and garnish

sea salt and pepper to taste

Option (okay for gut repair)
2 cloves minced garlic

Preparation

- Preheat oven to 400°F. Oil the bottom of a 9 x 13-inch (about 23 x 33 cm) baking dish with a lid.
- Rinse the salmon, and pat dry with paper towels. Sprinkle with salt and pepper, and place in the prepared dish.

- Mix the oil or ghee (if it is solid, then melt it on the stove top or on low in your toaster oven), lemon zest, dill, and optional garlic, and place about half the mixture on top of the seasoned salmon—you can spread the lemon dill mixture or leave it in dollops.
- Bake for about 20 minutes, depending on the thickness of the salmon, your altitude, and your oven. The salmon will continue cooking even after you take it out of the oven. Check on it every 10 minutes while it's baking.
- Top with the remaining oil, dill, and lemon zest mixture, add a squeeze of lemon juice, and serve with lemon slices and dill for garnish.

Tuna Stew with a Latin Groove

This stew is a personal favorite. The Latin Groove is represented by plantains instead of potatoes. As your gut heals, you can add a dash of cayenne. If you are ketogenic, limit consumption. This is a transitional recipe, due to the starchy plantains. Remember to only purchase wild tuna, not farmed.

Ingredients

2 lbs/1 kg fresh tuna, rinsed and patted dry, and cut into 1-inch squares

3 Tbsp ghee or avocado oil

2 carrots, 1 minced, 1 chopped

1 zucchini/courgette, quartered lengthwise and then sliced

1 medium onion, minced

4 large cloves garlic, minced

1 bay leaf

3 cups/720 ml vegetable or chicken broth (make sure it's free of hydrolyzed yeast, which is MSG)

1 cup/240 ml dry white wine (the alcohol will cook away), or ½ cup/120 ml clam juice and ½ cup/120 ml water, or add 3 tbsp fish sauce, obtainable from Asian markets

¼ cup/15 g minced parsley for garnish

Options (okay for gut repair)

½ tsp saffron threads

2 plantains (see below)

Valuable Option

2 plantains (I prefer these to potatoes!) **or 2 lbs/1 kg sweet potatoes**

Options (not for gut repair)

1 medium-hot chili pepper (poblano or Anaheim), seeded and minced, or **½ tsp red pepper flakes, or a dash of cayenne pepper, or 1 red pepper,** seeded and minced. **Note:** peppers are nightshades and non-ketogenic; a dash of cayenne pepper may be okay!

Preparation

- Preheat oven to 350°F. Peel and then slice plantains lengthwise, place in covered baking dish, and top with a dollop of coconut oil. Bake for 30 minutes. After baking, cut into 1-inch-thick pieces. Set aside.
- Separately mince one carrot (and, if using them, the red pepper and chili) in a food processor, with a few quick hits on the pulse button. Chop the other carrot, the zucchini, and the onion.
- Heat oil in heavy casserole, and cook carrots for 5 minutes, then add zucchini, and onions (and red pepper and chili pepper, if using them). Stir, and cook about 10 minutes, or until soft. Add garlic, bay leaf, and plantain. Cook for 3 minutes while stirring.
- Add broth, wine, and saffron. Bring to a boil. Reduce heat, and cook, lightly covered, for 20 minutes.
- Add tuna, salting to taste. Stir to mix. Cook to desired rareness: 3–4 minutes for rare; 5–6 minutes for medium.
- Discard bay leaf, and transfer stew to serving bowl. Sprinkle with parsley, and serve immediately.

Beef with Broccoli and Garlic

This simple combination of ingredients is certain to make your palate sing! Consider adding organ meats in this particular recipe.

Ingredients

2 Tbsp coconut or avocado oil or ghee

5 cloves garlic, minced

2 Tbsp ginger, peeled and minced

1–2 lbs/500 g–1 kg beef, cut into 1-inch cubes (Ask your local butcher for the best cut). You can also add organ meats

4–6 cups broccoli florets with some peeled and sliced stalks

½ cup/50 g green onions, thinly sliced

¼ cup/60 ml coconut aminos

sea salt and pepper to taste

Option (not for gut repair)

1 pepper

1 tsp red pepper flakes

toasted sesame seed oil instead of coconut oil, if you aren't being strict on gut repair or are mostly repaired and have been tested for cross-reactive foods and know that sesame is safe for you.

1 Tbsp white sesame seeds, for garnish

Preparation

- Heat coconut oil in a wok or skillet over high heat. Add garlic and ginger, and sauté for 2 minutes until oil is infused.
- Add steak, stirring until browned on all sides.
- When steak is seared, add broccoli. Continue to sauté over high heat. Add green onion. Add an extra Tbsp of oil, if needed.
- Add coconut aminos, and season with salt (and optional pepper and red pepper flakes). Continue to sauté another 2–3 minutes, until all the flavors are combined.
- Garnish with a sprinkle of sesame seeds or a sliver of raw garlic (optional).

Ginger Chicken with Broccoli

Ingredients

2–3 Tbsp coconut oil or avocado oil or butter/ghee

1–2 lbs/500 g–1 kg chicken thighs, cut into 1-inch cubes

4–6/500–750 g cups broccoli florets

½ cup/50 g green onions, thinly sliced

5 cloves garlic, minced

2 Tbsp ginger, minced

¼ cup/60 ml coconut aminos

salt and pepper to taste

Optional (after 2 months of gut repair)**: 1 tsp red pepper flakes**

Preparation

- In a wok or skillet, heat oil over high heat. Add garlic and ginger, and sauté for 2 minutes until oil is infused.
- Add chicken, stirring until almost cooked all the way through. Once chicken is almost done, add broccoli. Continue to sauté over high heat.
- Add green onion, and an extra tablespoon of oil, if needed.
- Add coconut aminos, and season with salt and pepper. Continue to sauté another 2–3 minutes, until all the flavors are combined. Serve warm.

Moroccan Lamb Tagine

I first discovered this recipe in the South of France and have created a low-maintenance crockpot version. I have never gone wrong serving this to guests! Make extra servings, because it is extraordinary for leftovers, when the herbs have seasoned the meat even more. Enjoy the higher ketogenic fat content. The ginger and turmeric help with digestion. Taking bitters or half a glass of kombucha may aid your digestion with this.

Ingredients

1 Tbsp avocado or coconut oil or ghee (lactose- and casein-free); more if needed

8 small French lamb shanks or a 3–4-lb/1.5–2 Kg leg of lamb, whole or cubed (ask the butcher to cube it; I often find a leg of lamb without bone and cube it myself)

1 Spanish or yellow onion, chopped

2 cloves garlic, sliced

1 Tbsp ginger, peeled and grated or minced

1–2 tsp turmeric powder or peeled and minced root

1 tsp ground cumin

1–2 cinnamon sticks, about 3 inches long

4 kaffir lime leaves

1 cup/150 g broccoli florets chopped into small pieces

2 cups/500 ml chicken stock or filtered water

1 sweet potato, not peeled, chopped

1 small butternut squash, not peeled, seeded and cubed (decrease or omit if strict ketogenic)

3–4 cups/750 g–1 Kg Cauliflower Rice (see earlier preparation method), on which to serve the stew

Option (okay for gut repair)

4 tsp fish sauce

1 carrot, sliced at an angle

Options (not for gut repair)

1 tsp chili or cayenne powder

1 tsp cardamom pods (about 4–6 pods)

4 large ripe tomatoes, roughly chopped

Preparation

Note: You can place all ingredients into a crockpot and cook on low for 6 hours or high for 3. Alternatively, you can prepare as follows.

- Preheat oven to 315°F.
- Heat oil in frying pan on high heat. Add the lamb, and cook for 2 minutes, browning each side. Remove and place in baking dish.
- Reduce heat in frying pan, add onions, and cook for 5 minutes.
- Add garlic and ginger, and cook 1 minute; then add optional chili, optional cardamom, turmeric, cumin, and cinnamon. Cook 2 minutes.
- Add fish sauce, kaffir lime leaves, optional tomatoes, and stock or water and bring to a boil. Remove from heat.
- Add sweet potatoes and butternut squash to baking dish with lamb. Pour sauce on top, cover and bake for 2 hours, or until lamb is tender or falling away from the bone, if you used shanks.
- Serve with Cauliflower Rice or on a bed of fresh, organic baby spinach.

Crockpot Chicken

This is the perfect recipe for working parents, busy healthcare providers, or late-night executives. You can start it before work and arrive home to a fully cooked meal, often with leftovers for lunch the following day.

Ingredients

1 whole chicken
¼ cup/15 g of rosemary, dried or fresh (a small handful of sprigs)
2 Tbsp sage leaves, dried or fresh

1 Tbsp tarragon, dried or fresh
1 Tbsp thyme, dried or fresh
sea salt to taste
½ cup/120 ml filtered water

Options (okay for gut repair, though higher in carbohydrates and not ideal in large amounts for ketogenic plan)

carrots, cut diagonally in 2–3-inch chunks
parsnips, cut as the carrots
acorn squash, seeded and cubed (peeling is optional)

butternut squash, not peeled, seeded and cubed
sweet potato, not peeled, chopped

Preparation

- Remove giblets, if there are any, add to a small pot of water, and cook until done. Place entire chicken, breasts down, in crockpot. Put the herbs inside the chicken, saving a small quantity of each to sprinkle on top. If using veggies, place them around and on top of the chicken in the crockpot. They will be very soft and tasty when done.

- Add water to crockpot, and cover with lid. Turn crockpot to High, or 325°F, and cook for 5–8 hours.
- Carve chicken, and serve with optional veggies and cooking juices, along with a side of gently stir-fried greens, if you like. We carve the entire chicken and save leftovers to add atop our salad the next day or to make lettuce wraps. Save the carcass for homemade stock.

Fish Tacos with Cream Sauce on Lettuce Wrap

This recipe can be made gut repair-friendly by omitting the cashews. Otherwise, it's considered a transitional recipe. If you are still including nuts, then it can work for you as is. Strict gut repair will omit the soaked cashews and replace with an extra avocado as well as ½ cup/120 ml of full-fat coconut milk or coconut cream to make the sauce. It's delicious either way.

Ingredients

¼ **purple cabbage,** shredded
1 small jicama, peeled and grated
1 carrot, shredded
1 red onion, diced
4 limes, juiced
1 head romaine or butter lettuce, washed and separated

1 Tbsp grapeseed or avocado oil
1½ lbs/750 g grouper, snapper, mahi mahi, or other white fish
½ bunch fresh cilantro, chopped
2 tsp cumin
2 tsp garlic powder

Optional (depending on gut repair)

2 red, orange, or yellow bell peppers, sliced or diced
1 tsp cayenne or chipotle pepper

Avocado Cream Sauce

¼ **cup/35 g soaked cashews** (omit for gut repair, and replace with ½ cup/120 ml full-fat coconut milk)

⅓ cup/80 ml lime juice
2 cloves garlic
¼ **tsp salt**

2 ripe avocados (add 1 more
avocado if omitting cashews)

Water to blend

Option (not gut repair-friendly for the first 2–4 months)
1 jalapeño, chopped

Preparation

- Prepare all of the vegetables. In a medium bowl, toss the cabbage, jicama, shredded carrot, and cilantro with the lime juice. Set aside.
- Chop the fish into bite-sized pieces, and place in a shallow dish.
- In a small bowl, mix the cumin and garlic powder (and cayenne or chipotle pepper, if desired). Sprinkle the spice mix evenly over the fish, and set it aside to marinate.
- Next, make the Avocado Cream Sauce by adding the cashews (or coconut milk and extra avocado), lime juice, garlic, salt, and jalapeño (optional) to a high-powered blender and blending well. Add only enough water to facilitate blending. Add the avocados and purée. Transfer the sauce to a serving bowl.
- Heat a medium-size skillet over medium heat. Add the grapeseed oil and then the fish. Cover and cook 5–7 minutes, stirring every few minutes to ensure the fish is cooked on all sides. Remove the fish to a serving bowl.
- To construct the tacos, start with a lettuce leaf, add fish and veggie toppings, and finish with Avocado Cream Sauce. Serve warm.

Baked Salmon with Herbed Crust

Ingredients

2 salmon fillets, about
5 oz/140 g each
3 Tbsp flax seeds, ground
2 tsp basil, dried
2 tsp oregano, dried
2 tsp rosemary, dried

2 clove garlic, minced
2 lemons—1 for zesting, 1 cut into
wedges for serving
1 Tbsp avocado oil
sea salt and pepper to taste

Optional (not gut repair-friendly for the first 2 months)
¼ cup/30 g macadamia nuts, almonds, or sunflower seeds, very
coarsely ground

Preparation
- Preheat oven to 375°F.
- Combine the ground flax seeds, optional ground nuts, herbs, garlic, lemon zest, and oil in a bowl to make the topping, then season with salt and pepper.
- Place the salmon in a glass baking dish, and spread the flax seed mixture over the top of the fish. Bake the salmon in the oven until the flesh is flaky and the crust is golden brown; avoid overcooking.
- Serve warm with lemon wedges and a salad, or over a bed of spinach.

White Fish with Lemon Tarragon Sauce

This is a wonderfully light dish. You may substitute orange for lemon, and it's still brilliant. It makes for a fabulous spring or summer meal, with a lovely side salad, stir-fried greens, or asparagus.

Ingredients

2½ lbs/55 g white fish, skin and bones removed

3 Tbsp fresh lemon juice

3 Tbsp fresh or dried tarragon leaves

¼ cup/1.2 Kg ghee (lactose- and casein-free) or avocado or coconut oil (look for an expeller-pressed oil with no coconut flavor), more if needed

dash of salt and pepper

Options (okay for gut repair)
Use **orange** instead of lemon, and add **½ tsp of orange zest** to sauce
½ cup/20 ml coconut milk (adds a lovely texture and flavor)
Bake and garnish with **a few capers**

Preparation
- Preheat oven to 325°F (if using a thicker white fish like halibut, increase to 350°F). Combine all ingredients except fish in blender or food processor, and blend well.
- Place fish side by side in a glass or ceramic baking dish, cover with sauce, and cover with a lid. Bake for 30–40 minutes, or until fish is tender and flaky.
- Serve on a bed of gently wilted (steamed) spinach or cauliflower rice or both!

Favorite Keto Breakfast

My husband calls this dish his FB, as in "favorite breakfast." It's a wonderful dish that can be made in a large batch, reheated on the stove top, and eaten any time of day, not just breakfast. The large quantity and wide variety of vegetables ensures that you're receiving multiple servings of a healthy rainbow of phyto (plant-based) nutrients at one sitting. A serving size is equal to the size of your clenched fist. If you are strictly keto, then omit the carrots, beets, and squash as they are likely too high in carbohydrates for you at this time. The elk meat is delicious and lean, but if you can't get elk or bison, you can substitute ground turkey or beef. This is an alkalizing, power-packed, simple meal that merely requires some chopping.

Ingredients

Everything but the kitchen sink! All veggies are optional.

- 1–2 lbs/500 g–1 Kg elk, beef, turkey, or bison meat, ground
- 4–5 tbsp coconut or avocado oil, duck fat, or ghee (lactose- and casein-free)
- 2–3 carrots, cut on the diagonal or quartered lengthwise and chopped
- 1 onion, chopped, or 3 green onions, whole thing chopped
- 2–3 large cloves garlic, minced (more if you love garlic)
- 1 parsnip, chopped
- 1 zucchini /courgette (or other summer squash), chopped
- 1 cup/150 g cauliflower florets
- 1–2 cups/150–300 g broccoli florets
- 5–10 stalks of asparagus, bottoms snapped off and then chopped into 1-inch pieces
- 3–4 kale leaves, chopped
- 3–4 dandelion leaves, chopped
- 3 large collard green leaves, include stalk if you wish, chopped
- 4 chard leaves (green or rainbow), chopped
- ½–1-inch/1.2–2.5 cm ginger, peeled and diced
- ½–1-inch/1.2–2.5 cm turmeric root, peeled and diced
- splash of coconut aminos or to taste (add to individual servings to avoid cooking the aminos)
- ½ cup/30 g parsley or to taste, chopped
- 1–2 Tbsp oregano, dried or fresh
- 1–2 Tbsp thyme, dried or fresh
- 1–2 Tbsp rosemary, dried or fresh
- 1 Tbsp sage, dried or fresh
- ¼ cup/15 g fresh basil, chiffonade style

Note: The spices are optional and can be mixed and matched.

Preparation

- Heat 1 Tbsp oil or fat in a skillet on medium heat. Cook the ground elk (or other meat) until done. Set aside.
- Chop and dice all veggies. Keep the leafy greens in a separate bowl. Chop them perpendicular to the stalk and then make several cuts along the stalk to shorten the pieces.
- Add 2–3 Tbsp oil or fat to a large, deep wok or pan. Add the onion and cook for 5 minutes. Next add the firmer veggies, such as carrots, asparagus, broccoli, ginger, turmeric, parsnip, and cauliflower, and cook for 5 minutes. Add the softer veggies, such as summer squash (zucchini, etc.).
- Add the cooked ground elk (or other meat), and stir to incorporate well.
- Add all the leafy greens, and stir. You may need to add more oil. I also cover for about 5 minutes and let the greens become slightly steamed and bright green. Cook longer for softer veggies.
- Remove from stove, and serve immediately. Consider topping with sliced avocados.
- Store in a sealed container, and reheat any time of day for a power-packed meal.

Thai Curry Beef and Sausage

This dish is delicious and relatively simple. Serve with Cauliflower Rice (see recipe in this book). Kaffir lime leaves can be found in most Middle Eastern markets and the freezer section of Asian markets as well. I use my homemade chicken broth from this book and turkey Andouille sausage.

Ingredients

2–3 Tbsp curry paste (red, green, panang, or massaman all work well). Some pastes contain chili peppers—not officially gut repair—but it's a tiny amount and may be acceptable to most healthcare providers and GI tracts. Otherwise use curry or turmeric powder.

1 can coconut milk, unshaken
2 cloves garlic, minced
2 small onions, sliced or diced (yellow or white)
3 cups chicken broth
1 yellow squash, sliced into round chunks
2 cups broccoli florets
1 zucchini, cubed or julienned

2 **carrots,** chopped at an angle

2–3 **kaffir lime leaves**

1 **lb/500 g beef,** cubed

1 **lb/500 g Andouille sausage,** sliced (I prefer turkey or buffalo)

½ **cup/30 g Thai basil leaves or any basil,** chiffonade style

4 **cups/600 g of Cauliflower Rice,** which can be sautéed in 2 tsp of fish sauce for this recipe (see Cauliflower Rice recipe)

Preparation

- Put curry paste into a large cast-iron or enamel-coated, oven-friendly pot and heat on the stove. It will become fragrant but not burn.
- Add ½ can/120 ml coconut milk, mostly the thick stuff from the top of the can, the cream. Incorporate well into the paste.
- When lumps are gone, add garlic and onions and the remaining coconut milk. Stir well until onions are soft.
- Add chicken broth, beef cubes, sausage, and kaffir leaves, and simmer 20 minutes.
- Add squash, broccoli, zucchini, carrots, and basil, and simmer for 10–15 minutes.
- Serve over Cauliflower Rice, and garnish with a basil leaf or two.

Keto Duck Surprise

This duck recipe is scrumptious. It's great for a ketogenic nutritional plan, providing fat from the juicy duck meat. Duck breasts are often small, so I recommend doubling this recipe and having it for lunch the next day. The extra day allows the spices to infuse the duck even more.

Ingredients

2 **duck breasts** (if you roast the whole duck, simply double your spices)

1 **Tbsp cinnamon**

dash of nutmeg

1 **tsp turmeric powder**

2 **star anise,** ground

1½ **tsp ginger powder**

¼ **tsp clove powder**

1 **tsp lemon peel,** either dried and ground or fresh zest (you may also use orange)

1 **Tbsp fennel seed,** ground

3 **Tbsp avocado or coconut oil, duck fat, or ghee (lactose- and casein-free).** Add more as needed

Optional: ¼ cup/60 ml stock, if you need more liquid for the sauce. It depends on the quantity of duck you are preparing.

Option (not gut repair-friendly)
dash of cayenne, but only after you've done comprehensive gut repair for at least 2 months.

Preparation
- Preheat oven to 375° F.
- Grind the fennel seeds and star anise with a mortar and pestle until powdered. Score the duck breast two or three times.
- Mix all the spices, the stock, and the oil together, and coat the duck, filling the scored areas with the sauce. Allow to marinate for 1 hour.
- Bake duck, covered, for 1 hour, or until done. (I'm at high elevation, so my cooking time varies slightly). The duck should be tender.
- Serve on freshly steamed bok choy or other greens with a twist of lemon.

Super Salmon Patties

This is a favorite in our household. I always make extra for lunch the following day. It can be a little tricky at first to get the patties to hold together. Feel free to add more ground chia or coconut flour. It's a delicate balance of oil quantity, pan, and oil temperature, and how firmly you pack these patties together. The first batch always seems a little crumblier. Be patient, and remember it's an art form. Always use a splatter guard or lid. I heat up the pans with oil first, on medium or medium high, and then add the nicely formed patties. If they fall apart, their flavor will scatter beautifully over the soft bed of delicate baby spinach leaves, so don't worry! Just enjoy.

Ingredients

2 cans (15 oz/425 g each) canned salmon or 2 lbs/1 kg cooked salmon, chilled and de-boned

2 ribs celery, halved lengthwise and finely chopped

¼ cup/15 g fresh parsley, chopped

½ cup/50 g (about 3) green onions, finely chopped

1 small jar capers

½ cup/90 g ground chia seeds

½ cup/60 g coconut flour

2–3 Tbsp coconut aminos

1–2 large cloves of garlic, minced

1–2 Tbsp of alternative mayonnaise, soy and egg free (olive oil or grapeseed oil). Avoid canola oil.

3–4 Tbsp freshly chopped dill, or 2 Tbsp dried dill, and a little fresh dill for garnish

1 Tbsp cumin powder, more to taste depending on your palate

½ tsp celery salt

sea salt and freshly ground black pepper to taste

1 cup/220 g coconut oil for frying—you may do batches and need more oil

Option (okay for gut repair)
2 tsp turmeric, peeled and chopped

Options (not for gut repair)
¼ tsp cayenne

2 tsp paprika

3 Tbsp gluten-free Worcestershire sauce (the Wizard's brand has a dash of soy, or make your own!)

1 cup/230 g Raw Macadamia Nut Aioli Mayonnaise (see recipe opposite)

Preparation

- In a medium bowl, use a fork to flake the salmon. Add the celery, parsley, onions, optional aioli, coconut flour, ground chia seeds, capers, mayonnaise, optional Worcestershire sauce, coconut aminos, celery salt, garlic, optional cayenne, optional pepper, dill, cumin, and optional paprika. Combine thoroughly.
- Make patties from about ½ cup/110 g each of the mixture.
- Place patties on a plate, cover tightly, and refrigerate for at least an hour, or even overnight.
- In a large skillet or flat grill pan, heat some of the coconut oil over medium heat for your first batch.
- Gently place chilled patties in skillet, and cook until browned, about 5–7 minutes, then carefully flip and brown the other side. (I cook them in batches, using a mesh splatter guard.) The first batch is usually the crumbliest as the pan is still heating. Drain patties on paper towels, and serve on a bed of baby spinach with fresh dill as garnish.
- This recipe is simple to double, and leftovers are easily reheated in a toaster oven or ground up and mixed with fresh salad the next day. Often, I simply add one more can of salmon rather than a true doubling of it.
- Makes five generous servings, plus leftovers.

Raw Macadamia Nut Aioli Mayonnaise

This is not gut-repair friendly, but if you're healed and feel strong enough to handle nuts, this is delightful! Some people may be able to have this after two months of gut repair, so please consult with your healthcare provider.

Ingredients

1 cup/120 g macadamia nuts
¾ cup/180 ml water, or as needed

1 tsp minced garlic, or to taste; I usually just toss in 1–2 cloves
½ tsp sea salt, or to taste

Preparation

- Blend all ingredients into a smooth mayonnaise in the food processor, adding more water as needed to produce desired consistency.
- Can be stored for 4–5 days in a tightly lidded glass jar in the fridge, so make extra and use it as a dip with veggies!

Apricot and Thyme Baked Chicken

This dish is quite simply delicious. If you're tired of the same old boring baked chicken, this will treat your taste buds. You can choose the chunky or smooth sauce version. The alcohol in the wine cooks off, so it won't negatively impact your gut repair. This is a transitional recipe due to the fruit, so ketogenic people should only have 1 full cup/125 g of this dish at a time due to the fruit.

Ingredients

4 lbs/2 Kg organic chicken, breasts, or thighs, or a combination
2 Tbsp ghee, duck fat, or avocado or coconut oil
3–4 leeks, finely chopped
2 cups/260 g or 9 oz dried, sulfur-free apricots, finely chopped

1–2 Tbsp thyme, fresh or dried (I prefer heavier thyme for this dish)
salt and pepper to taste
½ lemon, zested
1 cup/60 g fresh parsley, chopped
1 cup/240 ml white wine
1 cup/240 ml homemade chicken stock or water

Options (not for gut repair)
chopped and toasted pecans (after two months of gut repair)
¼ **tsp approx. freshly grated nutmeg to taste**
⅛ **tsp cayenne**—if you dare!

Preparation

- Preheat oven to 400°F.
- Heat oil of your choice in saucepan on moderate heat, add leeks, and cook for 10 minutes or until soft.
- Stir in chopped apricots, optional pecans, thyme, salt, pepper, optional nutmeg, zest, and parsley. Remove from heat, and allow to cool for 10 minutes.
- You can keep it chunky, or you can add to food processor with ½ cup/120 ml broth and ½ cup/120 ml wine. (I do a combination of half liquefied and half chunky.) More liquid may be required to make the sauce; add a little at a time until desired consistency is reached. Do in batches as needed.
- Place chicken in roasting pan, and pour in remainder, if any, of white wine and broth. Next add leek and apricot mixture on top of chicken.
- Bake covered in oven for 1–1½ hours, or until chicken is fully cooked.
- Serve with steamed broccoli or any green vegetable of your choice.

Crockpot Curried Beef Stew

This crockpot stew is a one-dish wonder! It's simple to throw the ingredients into the crock, leave for work or play, and return to a beautifully cooked meal. It's a lovely winter dish and will warm people's hearts at any potluck. You can alter the vegetables to suit your palate as long as you stay within the gut-repair list. If you are ketogenic, then decrease or omit the sweet potatoes. This can also make a great transitional recipe if you add more root veggies or squash.

Ingredients

1½ **lbs/750 g cubed meat: chuck roast, cross rib roast, or lean stew beef**
½ **tsp thyme**
2 **large cloves garlic,** diced

1 **medium-large yellow onion, or more,** sliced or chopped (you can also add 1 cup /250 g small round pearl onions)

1½–3 tbsp curry powder (I love curry so add to taste)

1 large yam, or 2 smaller ones, or sweet potato

2–3 carrots, sliced diagonally

1 cup/150 g broccoli florets (optional)

1 summer squash, such as zucchini or yellow squash, cut into quarter pieces

2 cups/500 ml beef broth or water or chicken broth

1 tsp sea salt or to taste

¼ tsp fresh cracked pepper (I use tricolor)

Options (okay for gut repair)

1 cup/150 g organic peas (I make the legume exception here)

¼/15 g cup cilantro, chopped for garnish

Options (not for gut repair)

½ lb (approximately 2 large handfuls) green beans (I make the legume exception here)

½ tsp paprika

3–4 large tomatoes, chopped (or 28-oz/800 g can diced tomatoes)

½ cup/75 g shiitake mushrooms or my favorite local wild lobster mushrooms, sliced

Preparation

- Lightly cook meat in a slightly greased pan (with olive oil or coconut oil) with the optional paprika, thyme, and pepper. It doesn't need to be cooked all the way.
- While it's cooking, chop yam into rounds or quarters, chop onion, carrots, summer squash, and optional tomatoes, and save as much juice as you can. Dice garlic, cut tips off optional green beans, and cut them in half for easier eating.
- Place everything in the crockpot, add meat, then deglaze the meat-cooking pan by swishing the broth or 2 tsp of apple cider vinegar, or water, around the pan scraping up any remaining bits, pour this into the crockpot. If you need more liquid, add another cup/250–500 ml or two of broth or water. The veggies will create more juice as they cook.
- Cook on low for 4–5 hours or high for 3–4 hours. Longer won't hurt, but the yams may fall apart.
- Ladle into soup bowls, and sprinkle with fresh cilantro.

Cooking Variation: Cook meat with broth and herbs in crockpot for 2 hours, then add vegetables for another 2 hours. Sometimes I add the summer squash about 30 minutes before I serve to prevent overcooking.

Chicken with Sausage, Prunes, and Apples

I first discovered this recipe while living in the South of France, in the tiny village of Montolieu. I had rented a very old, well-kept, three-story home that had previously been one of the older bookstores in the town. (Montolieu is known as a petite village de livre, a small book village, as there are many sweet bookshops that line the cobblestone streets.) This recipe is incredibly delicious and will leave your guests begging for more! This is a transitional recipe due to the higher carbohydrate content of apples and prunes. If you're ketogenic, limit your portion to ¾ cup/150 g, and enjoy the savory flavors in the evening. Don't worry if you miss a step; you can't ruin this one. Just add whatever you missed, stir, and proceed. When I self-catered my wedding, this dish was one of our mains. It always receives rave reviews.

Ingredients

¼ cup/60 ml avocado, grapeseed, or coconut oil, or ghee

1 lb/500 g sweet Italian sausage (try turkey sausage, ground turkey, or buffalo sausages)

1 chicken, (deboned), or 2¼ lbs/ 1 kg boneless chicken thighs or breasts, cut into bite-sized pieces or left whole

½ cup/120 ml raspberry or regular balsamic vinegar (or pomegranate or fig)

¾ cup/180 ml chicken stock or boxed/canned organic chicken broth (remember to avoid any containing "natural flavors")

¾ cup/180 ml dry white wine

1 bay leaf

1½ tsp dried thyme

sea salt and fresh ground pepper to taste

1 cup/175 g pitted prunes, halved

10 cloves garlic, halved lengthwise

1½ Tbsp Dijon mustard

2 large tart apples, cored, and cut into 1-inch cubes (If you are ketogenic, decrease to 1 apple)

1 Tbsp fresh flat-leaf parsley, chopped

Preparation

- Preheat oven to 350°F.
- Heat oil in ovenproof casserole or Dutch oven with lid. Brown the sausage, remove with slotted spoon, and set aside.
- Brown chicken pieces in casserole, using sausage fat, and set them aside with sausage. Pour off most of the fat, add 4½ Tbsp of the

balsamic vinegar, and boil over medium heat, scraping up any brown bits. Then add the stock, wine, bay leaf, thyme, and salt and pepper. Cook 1 minute.

- Add prunes and garlic to casserole, and cook 1 minute. Then return sausage and chicken, mix gently with sauce, and cover pot. Transfer to oven, and bake for 40 minutes.
- Using slotted spoon, remove the chicken, sausage, and prunes to a heated serving platter, and keep warm if possible. Add the mustard and remaining 3 Tbsp balsamic vinegar to the casserole, and whisk well. You may need another Tbsp of vinegar.
- Add the apples, and cook over medium-low heat until the apples and garlic are just tender, 5–7 minutes. Spoon the sauce over the chicken and sausage, sprinkle with parsley, and serve hot.
- Makes about four portions, but it's easy to double.

Keto Rosemary and Turkey Bacon Chicken Kabobs

This is a great recipe for both family and company when you're in the mood to grill. All ages will enjoy the flavors. This is a heavy-protein meal, so pair it with a large salad or leafy greens. If you can't find turkey bacon you can substitute pork bacon after two months of gut repair.

Ingredients

4 skewers for grilling

4 slices of turkey bacon, fried in a little coconut oil or cooked in a pan. Some brands need very little cooking. If you can't find turkey you can use pork bacon.

1 lb boneless chicken thigh or breast meat, cubed

⅓ cup/160 ml cooking oil, avocado, grape seed, coconut, ghee, duck fat, etc.

3 Tbsp coconut aminos

1 Tbsp fresh rosemary, minced

1 tsp lemon juice

1 tsp fig balsamic vinegar (or any flavor balsamic you have)

¼ tsp ground black pepper or to taste

2 tsp sea salt

drizzle of olive oil as you serve the skewers

Preparation

- In a medium bowl, stir together the cooking oil, coconut aminos, rosemary, salt, lemon juice, balsamic vinegar, and pepper. Let stand for 5 minutes. Place chicken in the bowl, and stir to coat with the marinade. Cover and refrigerate for 30 minutes.

- Fry turkey bacon until cooked through.
- Preheat the grill for medium-high heat. Thread the end portion of one strip of bacon onto skewer so the rest of the strip is hanging down. Skewer on a piece of chicken; thread on the next portion of the bacon. Turn the skewer so that the long end of the bacon is again hanging down. Repeat this process of skewering and turning until the entire strip of bacon is threaded, using 4–5 chicken pieces. Then discard marinade. (You can bake the chicken with the marinade and then skewer to serve)
- Lightly oil the grill grate. Grill skewers for 8–12 minutes, or until the chicken is no longer pink in the center and the juices run clear.
- Serve on top of gently steamed or stir-fried leafy greens, such as collards, chard, and kale with a twist of lemon. Drizzle the chicken kabobs with olive oil before you serve them.

Grilled Chicken with Tangy Lime Marinade

This chicken dish is simple and very delicious. I bake it, but it could be grilled. This is a heart-healthy meal! Who thought Mexican food could be gut repair-friendly? It is now!

Ingredients

3 limes, juiced, and their zest kept separate

3 Tbsp and ¼ cup/60 ml avocado or coconut oil

3 Tbsp Dijon mustard

3 Tbsp coconut aminos

6 green onions (or one large yellow onion), chopped and set aside

4 cloves garlic, minced and set aside

½ cup/30 g basil, chopped, chiffonade style

½ cup/30 g cilantro, chopped, discard stems

salt and pepper to taste

3 lbs/1,5 kg boneless chicken thighs

Preparation

- Combine the zest and juice of 2 limes, about ⅔ of the total liquid and zest, ¼ cup/60 ml avocado or coconut oil, all the mustard, coconut aminos liquid, half the green onions OR the entire yellow onion, half the garlic cloves, and salt and pepper. Mix well.

- Place chicken in a shallow glass dish, and pour marinade over the chicken. Marinate for 30 minutes in the refrigerator.
- Preheat oven, grill or grill pan to 350°F.
- Bake chicken covered for 40 minutes or until fully cooked. Or grill for 7 minutes. If grilling, flip and cook until internal temperature reaches 170°F, then remove from grill and allow meat to rest.
- Meanwhile, combine juice and zest of the rest of the lime with 3 tbsp avocado or coconut oil, the remaining chopped onions and minced garlic cloves, and the basil and cilantro.
- Slice chicken into bite-sized pieces or strips, and pour sauce over top.
- Serve warm on a bed of Cauliflower Rice (see recipe in this book) and a few slices of fresh avocado.

Keto Turkey and Zucchini Sliders with Coconut Yogurt Sumac Sauce

Inspired by *Jerusalem: A Cookbook*
by Yotam Ottolenghi and Sami Tamimi

These sliders are incredible! You may wish to make extras. I've also made this recipe into meatballs, over a bed of greens, and topped with the delicious sumac sauce. You can be ketogenic or on a transitional nutritional plan and enjoy this recipe.

Ingredients

1 lb ground turkey
1 large zucchini/ courgette, coarsely grated (about 2 cups/300 g)
3 green onions, thinly sliced
½ cup/90 g ground chia seeds
2 Tbsp fresh mint, chopped
2 Tbsp fresh cilantro, chopped

2 cloves garlic, crushed
1 tsp ground cumin
1 tsp sea salt
½ tsp freshly ground black pepper
6 ½ Tbsp oil for searing; consider coconut, avocado, duck fat, ghee

Option

If you have completed 2 months of gut repair, or are using small amounts of dried fruit, you can add ½ **cup/80 g of currants** to the turkey burgers.

Option (not gut repair-friendly)

½ **tsp cayenne pepper** after 2 months of gut repair

Sumac Sauce

1 cup/240 ml coconut yogurt,
  plain

1 tsp lemon zest

1–2 Tbsp freshly squeezed lemon
  juice

1 small clove garlic, crushed

2 Tbsp olive oil

1 Tbsp sumac (Whole Foods or
  online)

½ tsp sea salt

¼ tsp freshly ground pepper

Preparation

- First make the sumac sauce by placing all ingredients in a small bowl. Stir well, and chill.
- Preheat oven to 425°F.
- In a large bowl, combine all the ingredients for the sliders or meatballs, except the oil for searing. Mix with your hands, and shape into 10 small burgers, each weighing about 1½ oz, or you can make smaller meatballs.
- Pour enough oil into a large frying pan to form a layer about ¹⁄₁₆-inch deep. Heat over medium heat until hot, then sear the meatballs in batches on all sides. Cook each batch about 4 minutes, adding oil as needed, until they are golden brown.
- Carefully transfer the sliders or meatballs to a baking sheet or into a Pyrex dish. Bake until just cooked through.
- Serve warm or room temperature, with the Sumac Sauce spooned over them or on the side.

Keto Zucchini Pizza Boats

Ingredients

3 large zucchinis /courgette
  (1 zucchini per person)

1 lb ground meat or chicken
  (I prefer fatty beef or buffalo
  for this)

¼ cup/35 g black and/or green
  olives of your choice, chopped

½ large jar of marinated (in
  brine, oil, or local seasonings)
  artichoke hearts, cut in quarters

¼ cup/15 g carrots, shredded

1 small yellow onion, chopped
  and sautéed

1–2 cloves garlic, chopped and
  sautéed with the onion

1 Tbsp oregano or more to taste

2–3 Tbsp fresh basil or more to taste, chiffonade-style

3 Tbsp oil (avocado, grapeseed)

1 Tbsp olive oil

sea salt to taste

Optional (Not gut repair-friendly for the first 2 months)

½ cup/35 g mushrooms sautéed with onions

½ red pepper, chopped

½ can Italian tomatoes with basil and oregano, diced

vegan cashew cheese

vegan mozzarella cheeze (contains tapioca)

Preparation

- Preheat oven to 400°F.

Pizza Filling

- Sauté ground meat in a pan until done. Set aside. Chop onions and garlic, and sauté in a pan using avocado or grapeseed oil. Quarter artichokes, and chop olives. Shred carrots, and chiffonade the basil.
- Combine all ingredients, including the meat, veggies, 2 tbsp avocado oil, oregano, and basil, but wait on the olive oil. Stir well.

Zucchini Boats Prep

- Cut each zucchini in half lengthways. Next, take a spoon and gently run through the middle, scooping out the center (where the seeds are located). Be careful not to scoop the spoon too deep, as you'll break the skin of the zucchini. The goal is to create a hollow space to put your fillings in.

Zucchini Boat Assembly

- On a lined and greased (with avocado oil) baking sheet, place prepped zucchini halves, hollow part facing up. (To help them lie flat on the pan, you can also cut a piece off the bottom of the "boat" to create a flat surface)
- Next, stuff each zucchini boat with your desired fillings and cover with tinfoil. Bake for 20–25 minutes, until zucchini is tender (but not mushy). Save the vegan cheese for last. Uncover for the last 4 minutes and turn the broiler on to brown the top.
- Enjoy immediately with an extra drizzle of olive oil, or store in the fridge and reheat via toaster oven or conventional oven.

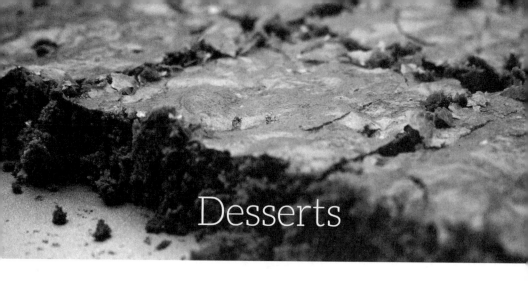

Desserts

Keto Coconut Butter Cups

Stick with coconut butter in the beginning; after 2 months of gut repair, you can try sunflower or another nut butter you like. This recipe is ketogenic supercharged, and will provide you with energy. You're going to want to double or even triple this recipe. Store them in the freezer, thaw them before consuming. Enjoy!

Ingredients

4 Tbsp raw cacao powder or toasted carob powder (cacao not gut-repair friendly for first 2 months)

4 Tbsp coconut oil or cacao butter

2 tsp Lo Han sweetener (monk fruit) or stevia leaf liquid to taste

4 tsp coconut butter, aka coconut manna

1 pinch sea salt

½ tsp raw vanilla powder or extract

Option

After 2 months of gut repair, you can use **cashew, sunflower, pecan, or hazelnut butter** instead of coconut butter.

Preparation

- Combine the coconut oil and cacao or toasted carob powder, Lo Han, and vanilla, and stir until there are no clumps. Add a pinch of salt to help bring out sweetness.
- If your coconut butter is not soft enough to spoon and pour, fill up a bowl with hot water and let the coconut butter jar sit in it for a few

minutes. You'll see the butter starting to become very soft along the edges of the jar. If it's winter, I remove chunks of coconut butter and heat on the stove on very low until it softens. Be careful not to burn it.

- Pour roughly half your chocolate mixture evenly into 4 metal, stone, or silicone cupcake molds sitting on a plate. (I've also used mini paper cupcake holders, and it worked perfectly, as they were just the right bite size and yielded more.)
- Tilt each cupcake mold around so that the chocolate mixture coats the edges a little. This will help hide the white layer of coconut butter. (This method works very well with paper liners, but as silicone ones are very nonstick, you'll still see some coconut butter peeking out from the sides.)
- Place in freezer for about 15 minutes.
- When the bottom layer has hardened, spoon 1 tsp of coconut butter onto each mold. Tap the plate of cupcake molds on your counter a few times so that the coconut butter spreads out evenly and covers the whole chocolate layer. Place again in the freezer for a few minutes.
- Lastly, take the remaining chocolate mixture, and cover the hardened coconut butter. Freeze one last time for about 15 more minutes.

I suggest doubling this recipe. Enjoy!

Raw Pumpkin Spice Cookies

Gut repair cookies—Yippeee!

Ingredients

½ cup/110 g coconut butter or coconut cream concentrate
1 cup/240 g pumpkin purée
¾ tsp ground ginger
¼ tsp ground cloves

¼ tsp ground cinnamon
1 tsp liquid vanilla or raw powdered vanilla
5 drops of stevia, or to taste

Options (not for gut repair)

¾ tsp ground nutmeg (this tiny bit is okay for gut repair)
¼ tsp ground cardamom
¼ tsp allspice
stevia to taste, or Lo Han fruit powder (monk fruit). If you're making it for guests you can consider using 1 tbsp coconut syrup/nectar, but not for gut repair for the first 2 months.

Preparation

- Thoroughly mix all ingredients in a bowl or food processor.
- Don't use the fruit roll sheets that most likely came with your dehydrator and fit on top of the tray; rather, cut parchment paper, and place it on your dehydrator trays—for some reason, the roll sheets prevent these cookies from drying properly.
- Drop heaping spoons of batter (about 2 Tbsp per cookie) onto parchment paper, aiming for 12 cookies per batch. Flatten the blobs of batter with the back of a spoon or rubber spatula until the cookies are about 2 inches/5 cm in diameter and about ½ inch/ 1.3 cm thick.
- Dry for 12–18 hours, until cookies are slightly crisp on the outside and cakey inside; dry longer for a crisper cookie. Remove the cookies after 10–12 hours, and place them directly on the dehydrator tray for a few more hours so the bottom dries more evenly.

Option

- Top the cookies with raw coconut meringue, or make mini sandwich cookies with the meringue in the middle.

10-Minute Keto Pumpkin Pudding

This recipe is very simple and fast to whip together, but it does need time to set. As the season changes from summer to fall, I'm inspired to make more warming dishes. As the October winds begin to blow, I often reach for pumpkin. In Traditional Chinese Medicine, pumpkin is cooling in nature and sweet and slightly bitter in flavor. The warming spices in this recipe balance the cooling nature of the pumpkin.

Ingredients

1 can (15 oz/420 g) organic pumpkin purée

1 can (15 oz/420 g) coconut milk, or substitute 1 cup/ 240 ml water

2 tsp kudzu root, dissolved in 2 tbsp water

3 tsp agar-agar flakes

2 tsp vanilla extract

2 tsp cinnamon

1 tsp powdered ginger

½ tsp clove

dash of sea salt

24 drops liquid stevia, vanilla crème flavor (quantity may vary, depending on brand)

Preparation

- In a medium saucepan, on medium heat, warm coconut milk (or water), and add agar flakes, stirring often. Bring to a boil for 2 minutes.
- Dissolve kudzu root in water, and add to boiling coconut milk and agar flakes. Lower heat, and simmer for 4 minutes, stirring frequently.
- Turn off heat, and add can of pumpkin purée, vanilla, and spices, and whisk together.
- Place in food processor, and blend all ingredients well. Immediately ladle into dessert dishes, and allow to cool on countertop for 10 minutes.
- Cover with plastic wrap, and refrigerate for at least 3 hours. Refrigerating overnight will allow the spices to fully integrate into the pumpkin.
- Top with Coconut Meringue or Coconut Cream recipes from this book, and enjoy!

Variation (not for gut repair)

After you've repaired your gut for a few months, you may begin to incorporate small amounts of specialty foods, such as **raw chocolate and carob**. Melt a little coconut oil with medium-roasted carob or cacao powder until desired consistency. Drizzle melted cacao or carob mixture over pudding. Refrigerate for another hour to allow to set. Garnish with a sprinkle of cinnamon, pinch of cacao powder, grated dark chocolate pieces, or raw cacao nibs.

Keto Chia Pudding

This healthy pudding is certain to put a smile on your face. You can have it for a snack or dessert. The chia seeds support your healthy colon and bowel movements, while the fat from the coconut milk offers you the energy you desire on a ketogenic nutritional plan. I often double the recipe.

Ingredients

1 can full-fat coconut milk
½+ cup/90+ g chia seeds
1 tsp cinnamon or to taste
1 tsp raw vanilla powder and or vanilla extract (do it to taste)

5 drops stevia or monk fruit or to taste (I prefer nothing as a sweetener for this one)
You may add ¼ cup/60 ml more liquid if you want it less thick

Options (gut repair-friendly)

1 scoop of protein powder (I like to use a vanilla-flavored pea protein powder or 1 Tbsp of beef collagen powder)
2 Tbsp medium-roasted carob powder

After 2 months of gut repair, you can use: **2 Tbsp raw cacao powder** and other milk substitutes, such as **almond, Brazil, hazelnut, or hemp,** contingent upon food sensitivities and cross-reactivity to foods.

Preparation

- Empty and scrape out coconut milk can, and blend coconut milk well by hand to incorporate any fat that collected at the top. Add chia seeds, and incorporate thoroughly. Add spices, stevia, optional protein powder, and cacao or carob powders, and stir well—consider using a whisk to make sure everything is thoroughly blended.
- Place in a shallow Pyrex glass dish, and refrigerate for 1–2 hours. The chia seeds will thicken the mixture into a luscious pudding.
- Serve with fresh organic raspberries, strawberries, blueberries, or blackberries. This makes a good dessert, or enjoy a few spoonfuls throughout the day as a tasty snack.
- Stores well in the fridge for about 1 week. Can also be frozen.

Raw Coconut Meringue

Inspired by *Sweet Gratitude: A New World of Raw Desserts* by Matthew Rogers and Tiziana Alipo Tamborra

This meringue is incredible! It's slightly more labor-intensive than the coconut cream on p. 235, but worth every moment. Make extra, as you're going to want it on top of everything. If you follow my step-by-step directions, you will be rewarded with scrumptious success!

Ingredients

¼ cup/60 ml coconut water or filtered water
¼–½ cup/60–120 ml coconut milk (regular not light, or blend coconut meat with its water)

1 cup/240 ml coconut milk
¼ cup/55 g coconut meat (double if you aren't using the soaked-cashew variation)
½ Tbsp vanilla

1 tsp lemon juice

⅛ tsp sea salt

1 Tbsp lecithin

½ cup/120 ml coconut oil

¾ oz/20 g Irish moss (see below)

Option (not for gut repair)

½ cup/60 g (dry weight) soaked cashews (use after 2 months of gut repair, or consult your healthcare provider. **Note:** make sure you aren't sensitive to cashews or cashew vicilin on the Cyrex Array 10)

Preparation

- Blend Irish moss (below) with water. Add coconut milk. Blend thoroughly.
- Add coconut meat, vanilla, lemon juice, and salt. Blend until smooth and creamy.
- Add lecithin (if you have an allergy to lecithin, omit and add 2 Tbsp more coconut oil)
- Pour into container, and refrigerate until slightly firm. I like to whip the meringue just before using it to help it fluff. Then I spread it on raw key lime pie, or raw pumpkin spice cookies, or use it to dip strawberries.

Irish Moss Preparation

- Irish moss can be found on the internet and in some raw cafés and specialty stores. If possible, get the kind still covered with sand and salt. This is normal, and there will be no lingering odor or flavor when processed properly.
- It's important to properly rinse and soak the Irish moss. Soaking according to these directions will yield moss that will last for 1 week in a sealed container in your refrigerator. Only soak what you'll use in one week. Unsoaked Irish moss, sealed and refrigerated, will last for months.
- Thoroughly rinse small amounts of Irish moss in cold water only (using warm or hot water will decrease the mucilaginous properties and render it less effective). Rinse the moss, one piece at a time, under cold running water. Place the rinsed pieces in a container, and fill with water. Mix the moss with your hands in the container, or seal the container and shake vigorously to release more impurities. Drain the water, and repeat 2–3 times, until the drained water is clear.
- Next, fill the container with water, completely covering the Irish moss, seal the container, and place in the refrigerator for 24 hours. Do not rinse the moss after this soaking process and do not drain or replace the soaking water.
- Remove the amount of moss you need for the recipe. You can use a small kitchen scale to weigh it. It needs to be blended and broken

down very well. Coarsely chop. and add to a food processor, blender, or Vita-mix. Always blend the moss with the initial liquid noted in the recipe before adding other ingredients.

- Blend until mixture is smooth and jelly-like. There won't be many, if any, small visible pieces left. The amount of time needed for blending depends on your kitchen appliances and the sharpness of their blades.

Coconut Custard
Inspired by my friend Emily

This custard is fantastic! Adults and kids alike will be begging for more. I was originally introduced to a version of this recipe by my friend Emily, who was struggling to find a birthday dessert that was gut repair-friendly. She blazed the trail for me with this recipe. I tweaked the original by replacing starchy arrowroot with kudzu root, which is especially helpful for digestion as it soothes the stomach and intestines. I also omitted the cup of sugar it originally called for and replaced it with liquid stevia or monk fruit. The results are outstanding! Making this custard 1–2 full days before serving allows for the subtle spices to emerge beautifully.

Ingredients

2 cans (14 oz/400 g each) coconut milk, full fat, not light

2 Tbsp kudzu root powder (also may be chunky)

3 Tbsp water (to dissolve kudzu, add a tsp more water if necessary)

2 tsp agar-agar flakes, or 1 tsp agar powder

1 Tbsp fresh squeezed lemon juice

1 tsp powdered raw vanilla, from inside the bean (you can slice open a bean pod and scrape out the middle or purchase it already prepared)

2 tsp vanilla extract

1½–2 tsp cinnamon

dash of sea salt

13–18 drops liquid stevia, vanilla crème flavor

¾ cup/60 g shredded, unsweetened coconut flakes (omit if you want to keep a simple creamy texture, or add if you desire a bit of texture in your custard; I like it both ways)

Monk fruit or stevia to taste

Options (okay for gut repair)
dash of ginger root powder
½–¾ cup/45–70 g goji berries, (gut-repair friendly after two months)

Preparation
- Whisk together 3 tbsp water with kudzu, and set aside.
- In a large, heavy-bottom saucepan, whisk together 1 can coconut milk with agar. Bring to a boil on medium-high heat, whisking repeatedly. Allow to boil for about 1 minute, then turn heat down to medium-low.
- Whisk water and kudzu mixture again and immediately add to agar mixture on stove top. Whisk constantly for about 3 minutes.
- Pour in second can of coconut milk, lemon juice, stevia, cinnamon, vanilla powder, and vanilla extract, and whisk constantly. Cook until it thickens, about 5 minutes.
- Add optional goji berries (only after two months of gut repair).
- If it looks like it may boil over, lower heat. Scrape the sides and bottom of saucepan with whisk, as kudzu and agar can accumulate there.
- Remove from heat and immediately pour into ramekins or dessert bowls. Allow to cool on the countertop for approximately 15 minutes.
- Garnish with sprinkle of cinnamon, sprinkle of unsweetened coconut flakes, or larger unsweetened coconut chunks.
- Cover with plastic wrap, and refrigerate for at least 24 hours. The dessert will be ready after only 2 hours, but the spices need more time to permeate the custard. It can be saved for 5–7 days in refrigerator.
- Serve with fresh berries.

Coconut "Make-A-You-Crazy-For-Me" Cream

This coconut cream topping is rich, creamy, and mouth-watering.
I use it on top of pumpkin cookies, pumpkin pudding, raw
chocolate mousse, on its own, and so much more! You will
be in a cream-filled state of ecstasy—dare to share it!

Ingredients
2¼ cups/500 ml or so of fresh coconut milk (to make, use the meat of 2–3 young white coconuts—thicker meat is better but not necessary— and the water of either one or both, depending on how abundant it is. You can substitute a can of full-fat coconut milk, but fresh is ideal)

2 tsp liquid vanilla

⅛ tsp salt

2 Tbsp lecithin (optional but helps with consistency)

¾–1 cup/180–240 ml coconut oil (melted)

½–1 cup/120–240 ml coconut butter (melted)

Option (okay for gut repair)

½ cup/45 g goji berries, soaked and blended. It gives a lovely orangey-pink color. Or you can garnish with them. Gut-repair friendly after 2 months.

Preparation

- All watery and oily liquid ingredients must be warmed to similar temperatures. Cold coconut water/milk combined with warm coconut oil/butter will cause the oil/butter to curdle and yield a granular texture. Coconut oil/butter melts at 76°F, so a good temperature range for all ingredients is 80–90°F.
- Warm the coconut milk/water.
- Blend the coconut meat, the warm coconut milk/water, vanilla, and salt until smooth. This may take a few minutes. If using goji berries, add to blender with the coconut for a delightful flavor and orangey-pink color.
- Add the lecithin and the warm coconut oil/butter, and blend again until smooth and creamy.
- Pour into ramekins or dessert bowls. Refrigerate for 2 hours, or until it hardens.
- Serve topped with blueberries, raspberries, blackberries, and or strawberries, and a drizzle of lavender, fig, or raspberry balsamic vinegar.

Optional toppings (okay for gut repair)

coconut flakes

goji berries—okay for most gut-repair programs, but check with your healthcare provider to make sure it's right for you.

Italian balsamic vinegar drizzle (it's thick and scrumptious!)

drizzle of melted cacao butter mixed with raw cacao (or substitute raw carob powder mixed with coconut oil). You can use raw cacao powder or raw cacao paste. Melt 1 Tbsp cacao butter on low heat, and mix with 2 heaping Tbsp of cacao powder. You can add liquid stevia to taste if the cacao is too bitter. (Use cocoa after 2 months of gut repair only).

Option (not for gut repair)

You may add 1 tsp honey, coconut syrup, or Yacón syrup (a syrup made from the Yacón tuber indigenous to the Peruvian Andes) to sweeten the chocolate. Gut-repair friendly options are stevia and monk fruit.

Raw Chocolate Mousse

Do you have children or guests with a sweet tooth? Do you wish to wean them over to a healthier diet and lifestyle? Do you want a fast and nutritious dessert to serve your family? This dessert is for you! (Don't tell them that the main ingredient is avocado!)

Sweet chocolate pudding is the perfect dessert for any occasion. This is a transitional recipe due to the chocolate. After 2 months of gut repair, it's great! Consult your healthcare provider to determine if raw cacao—chocolate—can be part of your gut-repair program. It comes from a bean but is also loaded with antioxidants.

Note: If you've done Cyrex Array 4, and it showed that you have a cross-reactivity to chocolate, remember that the chocolate used for that test is *milk* chocolate; what we are using here is raw cacao with no dairy whatsoever. With rare exceptions, this should be fine.

Ingredients

4 large avocados

½ cup/50 g (or to taste) cacao paste or raw cacao powder. Cacao paste is an added bonus if you can obtain it. (Whole Foods Market now carries cacao paste, or you can buy it online. It comes as a brick, so it's really not a paste at room temperature.)

2 young coconuts, water and meat. If the meat is too thin, watery, and translucent, add another young coconut.

½ cup/120 ml coconut oil or an additional ¼ cup/60 ml cacao butter, or a mixture of both. I prefer both, but I want to give you options in case you can't procure it.

cacao butter (available online or in specialty stores—it comes as a brick or in solid chunks and smells heavenly, just like chocolate)

stevia drops or monk fruit (Lo Han) to taste for strict gut-repair plans; if not strict gut repair, then **¼–½ cup/60–120 ml or 85–170 g raw honey or coconut nectar (syrup) or Jerusalem artichoke syrup (to taste), or a combination of these.**

2 Tbsp (or more to taste) cacao nib powder or raw cacao powder (I grind my own from nibs. but it isn't as finely ground as store-bought raw cacao powder.) Check taste to see if you need more powder if you replaced it for paste.

pinch or two of Saigon cinnamon to taste

1–2 tsp raw vanilla powder

1 tsp vanilla liquid

Options (gut repair-friendly)

dash of cayenne (not normally part of gut repair, but just this once I give you permission)

1 Tbsp Mucuna powder (great for dopamine enhancement—happy neurotransmitters in your brain)

1 Tbsp toasted maca powder

1 Tbsp wheatgrass powder

½ cup/45 g soaked goji berries

Hint (only 1–2 drops!) of rosewater or rose essential oil

Hint of mint or orange essential oil

Vanilla-flavored stevia drops

Preparation

- Melt cacao paste on very low heat, preferably in a double boiler. While it's melting, add coconut oil or cacao butter. If you're using cacao powder instead of paste, simply melt with the coconut oil or cacao butter.
- Drain coconuts, scoop out meat, and save the liquid.
- Put avocados in food processor, and blend. Add young coconut meat and coconut water, and blend. Add honey or coconut nectar syrup (not gut repair) or stevia drops, and blend. Add cacao and coconut oil/cacao butter, and blend, until very rich and creamy. Add more sweetener, spices, or chocolate to taste.
- Dish into small serving bowls and refrigerate for 2 hours.
- Serve with Coconut Meringue or Coconut Cream (see recipes in this book) or fresh raspberries.

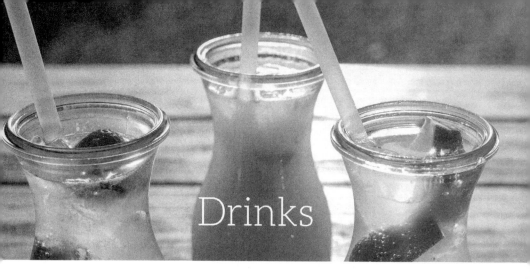

Drinks

Kombucha

Kombucha is a fermented beverage that smells like vinegar but tastes like a sparkling cider. It's been touted as a health elixir for at least 2,000 years, although there is little scientific research to date. I love the taste and believe that digestion improves when consumed around mealtimes. That said, I also want to share that my body no longer enjoys how it feels. So, in honor of my body, I no longer consume it. This is what I mean by being self-aware around food!

I have several favorite recipes, but the sky is the limit. At first glance, you may feel overwhelmed, but after the first few batches, you will get the hang of it and be thrilled with your results! Bring to a potluck, serve with dinner or dessert, keep it all to yourself, or host a kombucha tasting party in your neighborhood.

Note: You will need to purchase a starter known as a SCOBY (symbiotic culture of bacteria and yeast), a baby kombucha pad, in order to begin fermenting your kombucha.

Coconut Vanilla Kombucha

Ingredients

4-liter, lead-free glass jar (such as old olive or pickle jars)

4 liters filtered water

4–5 bags Republic of Tea Vanilla Coconut 100 percent White Tea, or other tea of your liking

2 raw vanilla pods, sliced down the middle

1½ cup/420 g raw sugar (sucanat)

cheesecloth

Option

When you bottle your tea, after following the entire preparation below, you can add 4 dried cherries to the bottle, along with the pinch of sugar. Now you have coconut, vanilla, cherry fizziness! Allow to sit in refrigerator for at least 4 days, but longer is better, before you consume.

Preparation

- Boil water with tea bags and vanilla pods. Allow to cool. When still warm, add the sugar, and stir well. When completely cooled, stir well and remove pods and tea bags with a slotted spoon.
- Pour into 4-liter glass jar. Cut cheesecloth to fit over top. Cut up old clean cotton tee-shirt or pillow case to fit over top of that. Place cheesecloth and then cotton cloth over top, and secure with large rubber band around mouth of jar.
- Keep in semi-dark to dark place, like a cabinet or pantry.
- The size of your SCOBY and air temperature will determine how fast your kombucha will ferment, so keep checking. If you have only one new SCOBY, it takes about 2 weeks. The SCOBY will grow, meaning the pad will produce multiple layers. The thicker it is, the quicker it ferments. Eventually you can gently peel off the lowest pad, and discard. If you wish to share with a friend, consider giving them a newer pad.
- You want the drink to be sour and slightly sweet, even a little fizzy. If it tastes like sweet tea it isn't ready. If it tastes like pure vinegar, it has gone too long and needs to be double fermented. You do this by dissolving 1½ cups/420 g sugar into 2 cups/500 ml warm water, then add to the vinegar liquid with the kombucha culture, and allow it to ferment again. This time check it sooner.
- When you harvest the liquid, always leave a little remaining, just covering your pad. When you bottle the liquid you harvested, add a few pinches of sugar before you cap it, and place in the fridge. Cut a bit of parchment paper, and place between the lid and the mouth of the bottle, then seal with the lid. Leave on your countertop for 24–72 hours to allow the anaerobic fermentation to occur. This will increase the fizziness while consuming the sugar. Store in the refrigerator.
- Enjoy morning or night, before, during, or after meals!

Pomegranate Kombucha

Ingredients

3 liters filtered water

4–5 bags of Republic of Tea Pomegranate Green Tea or other tea of your liking

1 cup/240 ml pure pomegranate juice

1 cup/280 g raw sugar (sucanat)

Preparation

- Boil water with teabags and cool, adding sugar when it's still warm.
- Follow preparation from previous recipe. This time add (uncooked) pomegranate juice directly into the jar with the SCOBY.

Ginger Hibiscus Kombucha

Ingredients

4 liters filtered water

4–5 bags of Tazo Passion herbal tea or other fruity tea

4–5 slices of ginger, about ½-inch or 1 cm thick

1½ cups/420 g raw sugar (sucanat)

Options

Cook pure hibiscus flowers (found dry in bulk sections of herb and health food stores) in a muslin bag, or simply strain out of tea. You can also leave in kombucha, but it's nice to rotate flavors, and you don't always want lingering flowers in the next batch.

Preparation

- Process same as above, and remove chunks of ginger, just as you removed the vanilla pods and tea bags, before adding tea to your large glass jar. Some people like to keep the ginger.

Cinnamon Rose Kombucha

Ingredients

4 liters filtered water

4 bags of Tulsi Cinnamon Rose Tea or other tea of your liking

1 heaping tbsp of rose hips in a tea ball or muslin bag (optional)

1 cinnamon stick

1½ cups/420 g raw sugar (sucanat)

Preparation

- As above. Remove rose hips, cinnamon stick, and tea bags before adding your tea to the jar.

The Best Strawberry Lemonade in the Universe
Inspired by my friend Pete

This is a transitional recipe and perfect for a hot summer day. Both adults and children can enjoy this refreshing drink. The lemon helps detoxify the liver and alkalize the body.

Ingredients

5 strawberries, fresh or frozen
1 lemon (squeezed)
5 oz/150 ml purified spring water

3 drops of stevia or monk fruit to taste (optional)

Variations

Cook **1 inch or 2.5 cm of sliced ginger root in water for 30 minutes,** allow to cool, then add other ingredients

Any fruit or combination of fruit, such as raspberries, can be substituted for strawberries

Lime can be substituted for lemon

Try adding **mint, rosemary, basil, or any other fun herbs or spices** you like. You could also use **food-grade essential oils** for ease and benefit if herbs aren't available.

Preparation

- Just blend, and serve!

Flavored Water

Are you tired of plain water? Here are a few tricks to help you drink more water! Essential oils are concentrated and therefore strong; fewer drops are better. Please make sure that your essential oils are food-grade and organic.

Ingredients

Choose ONE of the following or mix and match as you desire:

1 drop of peppermint essential oil

1 drop of spearmint essential oil
1 drop of fennel essential oil

1 drop of lemon or lime
essential oil

1 drop of orange essential oil
1 drop of ginger essential oil

Options

cucumber slices

lemon or lime twist

organic rose petals

1 Tbsp goji berries

2 drops of any flavored stevia
extract

mint leaves or sprigs (add to water
bottle, and leave for one day)

Lemon balm leaves or sprigs
(this is a TH1 stimulator, so
if you have an autoimmune
challenge, be aware of any
flare-ups after consuming it.
This small amount should be
fine, but everybody reacts
differently.)

Keto Peppermint Hot Chocolate

Ingredients

2 cups/500 ml coconut milk—
I prefer the thick, full-fat can of
coconut milk (after gut repair
you can also use almond or
cashew)

2 heaping tsp gluten-free
toasted carob powder

2 dashes of cinnamon

1 drop peppermint essential oil

¼ -1½ tsp of raw vanilla bean
powder; you can also scrape
the inside of a vanilla bean, or
add vanilla extract

5 drops stevia, or to taste (I like
vanilla crème flavor) or monk
fruit to taste

Optional (okay for gut repair)

Kudzu root is a healthy alternative thickener. It is great for digestion! Mix 1
heaping tsp into the milk alternative, and stir well for about 4 minutes on
high temperature, see below.

Optional (not gut repair-friendly for the first 2 months)

Substitute raw cacao powder for toasted carob.

Preparation

- Warm milk alternative on the stove, and add optional kudzu root, heat
to high, and stir well for 4 full minutes. If it starts to boil, then decrease
the temperature slightly, and keep stirring. If you aren't using kudzu
root, then heat the milk, and move to the final step.

- Next, add all other ingredients. and either whisk until blended, or use a hand blender to mix all the ingredients. I find that a hand blender helps the carob integrate with the milk better than a whisk. Serve warm and enjoy.

Dare to Be Green

This is my own famous green drink. I've had so many requests for it that I decided to include it in this book. It's a power-packed, perfect way to begin the day. I have it for breakfast several days a week and when I'm on the road, it's an easy travel food—I bring all the powders with me, add water, and enjoy. It's incredibly "green," and some may need to gradually work up to this alkalizing drink.

When educating patients and training their taste buds, I encourage them to add raw cacao powder, lemon/lime, or blueberries to help with flavor in the beginning. Depending on the person and how much they need to add dietary greens, I may even suggest a banana, but this has a lot of sugar and is not gut repair- or ketogenic-friendly but works to get greens into people who may desperately need them.

Ingredients

1 scoop grass-fed beef protein isolate, or 1 scoop collagen hydrolysate, or bone broth protein isolate, or pea protein, or beef protein hydrolysate. I often mix 1 scoop from two different products for a total of two scoops of a protein source. (See my section on Protein Powders in this book.)

2 tsp of a green food powder including spirulina and chlorella

1 Tbsp of a green food powder including kale, parsley, lemon, broccoli, beets, ginger, nettle, spinach, and dandelion or some combination of these

1 scoop of a green grass powder mixture including wheat, alfalfa, oat, and barley grasses

1 serving of a probiotic designed to be taken with food (Professional-quality powder is best. I prefer 100 billion CFU)

1–2 tsp of omega-3 oil and/or Arctic cod liver oil

½–1 cup/120–240 ml aloe vera
juice, whole leaf
½ cup/120 ml water or coconut
milk (canned coconut milk will
make it creamier)
1 Tbsp coconut oil

½ avocado
frozen açai berry powder packet,
slightly thawed (make sure it
is the unsweetened one. This
is safe for both gut repair and
staying ketogenic.)

Options

1 cup/240 ml coconut water
(after gut repair—it may kick
you out of ketosis if you do too
much, as it has high sugar)
½ cup/120 ml full-fat coconut
milk
1 Tbsp chia seeds, ground or
whole

2 tsp raw cacao powder (after
gut repair for 2 months)
1 tsp cinnamon
2 drops peppermint oil or to
taste
½ lemon, juiced (this can be
frozen in ice cube trays to add
slushiness)

Important Variations to Consider

If you aren't used to green drinks, keep it simple at first. Try the grasses
powder with berries, and see how your palate responds. Next add
spirulina and chlorella, beginning with ¼ tsp and working up, as it is very
detoxifying (may cause detox reactions like diarrhea). Increase by ¼ tsp
weekly or biweekly. Next add a whole-food green powder. Your taste
buds will change, and your mind—body—spirit will soar.

If you like it thicker, you can add ¼–½ cup/60–120 ml unsweetened
coconut kefir.

I have a friend who adds whole chia seeds to his green drink because he
likes to chew them. It will make the drink more gelatinous, so you'll want
to drink it right away.

Preparation

- Add all ingredients to a blender or hand mixer, and blend. Voilà! Drink
  immediately. When I travel internationally, I use a blender bottle, add
  ingredients, shake, and drink.

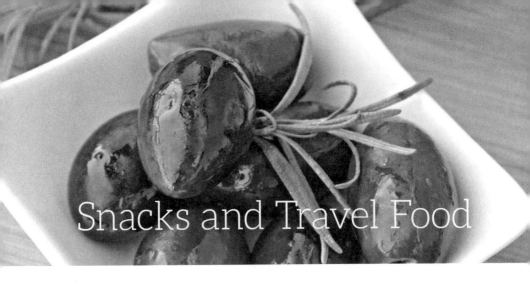

Snacks and Travel Food

Raw Kale Chips

It can be difficult to find a kale chip without nuts, so here it is.
These are a crunchy nutritious snack that both adults and kids love!

Note: I have included a nut option below that can be used once
your intensive gut-repair program has been successful and your
healthcare provider has proven, *through blood work,* that you
can have an occasional nut without an immune response. If
symptoms appear, return to the gut repair-friendly version.

Ingredients
2 bunches of curly kale (consider making a double batch; they go fast!)

Options (okay for gut repair)
1 zucchini/courgette, chopped
**1–2 Tbsp curry powder OR dried
    rosemary and 1 tsp of thyme**
    or other herbs to your liking
2 Tbsp chia seeds, ground

1–2 Tbsp fresh lemon juice to
    taste
sea salt and pepper to taste
2 Tbsp coconut aminos

Options (not for gut repair, but wowza!)
Add the ingredients above plus:
**1–1½ cups/120–180 g
    macadamia nuts**
1 red pepper
1 large tomato

⅛ tsp cayenne pepper
1 apple (if you are doing some
    fruit, this is a lovely addition)

Preparation

- Place all ingredients except the kale in a food processor, and blend into a semi-thick sauce. While blending, roughly chop the kale, and remove the stalk and thick parts of the vein, which harden like a stick when dehydrated.
- Pour the sauce all over the kale. Rub and mash the kale with the sauce so that all kale pieces have some sauce on them.
- Lay the kale on dehydrator trays, and dehydrate at 108°F for about 12 hours, or overnight. (If you don't have a dehydrator you can use your oven as long as it goes very low. Use the lowest temperature setting possible.)
- Store in an airtight container, and enjoy as a snack. They will last at least a week, depending on the humidity of your environment.

Raw Zucchini Chips

This simple, raw, crunchy snack is great with dips or alone. Several variations are listed below. The quantity varies depending on the size of your zucchinis. You'll need a dehydrator for this, or an oven in which you can keep the temperature very low. They shrivel, so make extra. The zucchini can be cut in thirds using a diagonal cut, then sliced in a food processor. The diagonal cuts make for a longer chip, which is useful when the zucchinis are small. I tend to fill 6–8 dehydrator trays' worth, and they hardly last 4 days.

Ingredients

4–10 zucchini/courgette (depending on size), sliced thinly into rounds about ⅛ inch or 1 cm thick

1 tsp sea salt

¼ cup/60 ml unrefined olive oil or melted coconut oil, enough to lightly coat but not saturate zucchini

Options (okay for gut repair)

1 Tbsp curry powder, sprinkled all over zucchini or mixed into oil

1 Tbsp rosemary, thyme, or any other herb you fancy

2 Tbsp coconut aminos or more to taste, depending on the quantity of zucchini

Preparation

- Slice zucchini, and place into a large deep bowl. Slice by hand or with slicing attachment on food processor for a more uniform look and feel, and shorter prep time.
- Add oil and herbs to a small bowl, and mix well. Incorporate into bowl with zucchini, coating the zucchini but not drenching them.
- Lay on dehydrator tray, side by side. Dehydrate at 108°F for about 12–48 hours or as high as 145°F for crunchier chips. This lower temperature helps retain vitamins and minerals. Times will vary depending on how much oil you use and the climate you live in. If your chips aren't crunchy, keep dehydrating them; you won't hurt them. They will crunch up a little bit more when they cool from the dehydrator.
- Enjoy with raw pesto, guacamole, or the Hearts of Palm Dip in this book!

Raw Rosemary Sweet Potato Chips

Need a crunch? These chips are a wonderful alternative to regular potato chips, and they make easy travel food. Sweet potatoes do not need to be cooked and are full of vitamins C and A, fiber, calcium, and potassium. They are starchy, so enjoy in moderation.

Ingredients

1 large sweet potato, sliced paper thin

2–4 Tbsp olive oil

1–2 Tbsp lemon juice

1–2 tsp dried rosemary, crushed or powdered

½–1 tsp sea salt

Preparation

- Use a mandoline slicer or the slicer attachment on your food processor to cut paper-thin slices of sweet potato. Put thin slices in a bowl, and gently coat with oil and lemon juice. Add salt and rosemary, and toss to combine well.
- Place slices on dehydrator trays, side by side. Dehydrate 6–12 hours at 108–145°F, or until crispy. The lower temperature will take a little longer but will keep enzymes active. The higher temperatures will speed the process.

Beef Jerky

Beef jerky is another of my favorite travel foods!
It's dried meat and is a great source of protein for a
quick travel snack, I bring this snack on long hikes,
backpacking trips, bike rides, and plane trips.

Two lbs of fresh meat will yield approximately 1 lb of jerky.
Thin London broil works well. Ask the butcher to cut into thin
strips for you. Let them know you're making jerky, and they will
cut it appropriately. Flap meat is another good cut for jerky, but
sometimes costs more. Skirt steak is a little more expensive
and a little fattier, which creates a more decadent jerky.

Ingredients

meat

sea salt, about 1–2 tsp per pound
of meat

drizzle of olive oil

Options (okay for gut repair if you're careful)

meat rub (check the ingredients to make sure it doesn't have gluten, soy,
sugar, paprika, MSG, or any other ingredients or spices that are not gut
friendly)

gluten-free Worcestershire sauce (fantastic, but some contain soy and
are therefore not good for gut repair)

curry powder (makes a wonderful jerky addition—use 1–2 tsp per pound
of meat)

2–3 Tbsp coconut aminos per pound of meat

Preparation

- Put strips of meat in a large metal, ceramic, or glass bowl. Add the
spices, sauce, and a drizzle of olive oil. Mix well, and allow to marinate in
the refrigerator for a few hours. The marinating police won't ticket you
if you don't, but the flavor will be improved if you do.
- Lay strips on dehydrator trays, and dehydrate at 108°F for about 12
hours. If meat strips are very thick, they may take 18 hours. I like certain
cuts of meat well done and crunchier for jerky, and others a little more
chewy. You'll discover what you prefer. It's always better to check it
early and then add more time, little by little, rather than making it too
crispy on your first try.

- If you're consuming immediately, it doesn't require any refrigeration. However, if you are traveling with it, refrigerate upon arrival to extend shelf life. Backpacking batches should be more well done, as refrigeration is often unavailable. If you're leaving it out on the counter, place it in a covered glass container. More humid climates will require refrigeration.

Young Coconuts

I first heard the inside of coconuts referred to as "jelly"
while traveling in the Bahamas. But I'm on an island, without
a machete of my own, so what's a coconut-lovin' woman to do?
Well, the island spirits were watching over me and led me to a
strong and beautiful French woman, Leo, who offered to bring
me some coconut "jelly." She had a very original way of cracking
them open, straight from her trees. She'd run them over with
her big-ass truck! Need I say more? I had enough coconut
jelly to keep me content for the remainder of my stay.

Wise Coconuts

It may be slightly labor-intensive until you get the hang of it,
but aged coconuts, the ones with the shaggy brown husk, are an
excellent snack and travel food! Feed your brain with a crunch!

Ingredients
1 wise coconut (aged, with brown husk)

Preparation
- A hammer and flathead screwdriver work well. Use the hammer to punch the screwdriver into one of the coconut eyes.
- Allow the water to drain into a measuring cup. If you find it isn't draining easily, make another hole in the adjacent eye.
- Take the empty coconut outside to a hard surface (like a concrete driveway), and crack it open with the hammer. Use the flathead screwdriver to pry the white meat away from the shell.

- Rinse the chunks, and refrigerate. It's perfectly fine to eat the thick brown skin that may stick to the white fleshy chunks as long as it's soft. Make certain to remove hard pieces of shell—a cracked tooth is never fun.

Note: Sometimes you may get a bad coconut. It won't smell right, or it may have purple spots or actual mold.

Wise coconut meat will last refrigerated for 5–7 days. It even lasts a good day or two without refrigeration, so makes great travel food. I have often brought it with me on the plane domestically, but you may not be able carry it when entering another country.

Canned Wild Sardines and Salmon

This is an easy travel food. I throw a few cans in my suitcase. It's a quick protein snack. I purchase them in olive oil with the bones, so I have the benefit of extra calcium; the bones are soft and easy to chew. I eat them on a salad or just out of the can. Make sure they're wild-caught.

Olives

Olives are a wonderful snack! If you haven't explored your local organic grocery store's olive bar, it's worth a peek. I used to occasionally eat olives from a jar but was never very impressed until I finally tried the olive bar. When serving yourself, add a little brine (the water the olives are sitting in) to retain color and flavor. If you don't have access to an olive bar, try various kinds in jars for a start. It's simple to whip up a homemade olive tapenade to dip your zucchini chips in. Be mindful of pits. Castelvetrano is my personal favorite. They are a bright green color with a buttery flavor.

Notes

1   Udo Erasmus, *Fats that Heal, Fats that Kill* (Alive Books, 2010), 416.

2   NIH, Autoimmune Diseases Coordinating Committee, *Autoimmune Diseases Research Plan*, 2006.

3   Corado Betterle, Zanchetta R, "Update on Autoimmune Polyendocrine Syndromes (APS)," *Acta Biomed* 74, no. 1 (April 2003): 9–33.

4   Amino N, "Autoimmunity and Hypothyroidism," *Baillieres Clin Endocrinol Metab.* 2, no. 3 (August 1988): 591–617.

5   Strieder TG, et al., "Risk Factors for and Prevalence of Thyroid Disorders in a Cross-Sectional Study Among Healthy Female Relatives of Patients with Autoimmune Thyroid Disease," *Clin Endocrinol (Oxf).*, 59, no. 3 (September 2003): 396–401.

6   Ley RE, Peterson DA, Gordon JI, "Ecological and Evolutionary Forces Shaping Microbial Diversity in the Human Intestine," *Cell*, 124, no. 4 (February 2006): 837-848. http://doi.org/10.1016/j.cell.2006.02.017.

7   Shulzhenko, Natalia, "Gut Microbes Closely Linked to Range of Health Issues," Oregon State University, accessed September 16, 2013, http://oregonstate.edu/ua/ncs/archives/2013/sep/gut-microbes-closely-linked-proper-immune-function-other-health-issues.

8   Bouskra D, Brézillon C, Bérard M, Werts C, Varona R, Boneca IG, Eberl G, "Lymphoid Tissue Genesis Induced by Commensals Through NOD1 Regulates Intestinal Homeostasis," *Nature*, 456, no. 7221 (November 2008): 507–510. https://doi.org/10.1038/nature07450.

9   Bouskra et al., "Lymphoid Tissue Genesis."

10 Salminen S, Bouley C, Boutron-Ruault MC, et al., "Functional Food Science and Gastrointestinal Physiology and Function," *British Journal of Nutrition,* 80, supp 1 (August 1998): S147–S171. https://doi.org/10.1079/BJN19980108.

11 Lierre Keith, *The Vegetarian Myth* (Oakland: PM Press, 2009): 40.

12 Keith, *Vegetarian Myth*, 9.

13 Zhou W, Mukherjee P, Kiebish MA, Markis WT, Mantis JG, Seyfried TN. *The calorically restricted ketogenic diet, an effective alternative therapy for malignant brain cancer.* Nutr Metab. London: 2007 Feb 21;4:5. https://www.ncbi.nlm.nih.gov/pubmed/17313687.

14 Gregory L. Austin, Christine B. Dalton, Yuming Hu, Carolyn B. Morris, Jane Hankins, Stephan R. Weinland, Eric C. Westman, William S. Yancy, Jr., and Douglas A. Drossman, "A Very Low-Carbohydrate Diet Improves Symptoms and Quality of Life in Diarrhea-Predominant

Irritable Bowel Syndrome," Clin Gastroenterol Hepatol. 2009 Jun; 7(6): 706–708.e1. https://www.ncbi.nlm.nih.gov/pmc/articles/PMC2693479/.

15 Stephen D. Phinney and Jeff S. Volek, *The Art and Science of Low Carbohydrate Performance* (Miami: Beyond Obesity LLC, 2012).

16 Phinney and Volek, *Low Carbohydrate Performance*, 11.

17 Ibid, 7.

18 Ibid, 10.

19 Henderson ST, "High Carbohydrate Diets and Alzheimer's Disease," *Med Hypotheses* 62, no. 5 (May 2004), 689–700. http://doi.org/10.1016 /j.mehy.2003.11.028.

20 Engelberg H, "Low Serum Cholesterol and Suicide," *Lancet*, 339, no. 8795 (March 1992): 727–728. https://doi.org/10.1016/j.mehy.2003.11.028.

21 Colpo, Anthony, *The Great Cholesterol Con: Why Everything You've Been Told About Cholesterol, Diet and Heart Disease Is Wrong!* (LULU, 2006), 26.

22 Longo VD & Mattson MP, "Fasting: Molecular Mechanisms and Clinical Applications," *Cell Metabolism* 19, no. 2 (Feb 2014): 181–92. http://www.ncbi.nlm.nih.gov/pubmed/24440038, https://doi.org /10.1016/j.cmet.2013.12.008.

23 Tel Aviv University, "How High Carbohydrate Foods Can Raise Risk for Heart Problems," *ScienceDaily*, June 27, 2009, accessed October 2, 2013, http://www.sciencedaily.com/releases/2009/06/090625133215.htm.

24 Cordain, Loren, and T. Colin Campbell, "The Protein Debate," *Performance Menu Journal of Nutrition & Athletic Excellence,* accessed March 8, 2015, http://www.catalystathletics.com/articles /downloads/proteinDebate.pdf.

25 Taubes, Gary, "What If It's All Been a Big Fat Lie?" *New York Times*, July 7, 2002, 5. http://www.nytimes.com/2002/07/07/magazine /what-if-it-s-all-been-a-big-fat-lie.html.

26 M. A. Sanjoaquin, P. N. Appleby, M. Thorogood, J. I. Mann & T J KeyNutrition, "Lifestyle and colorectal cancer incidence: a prospective investigation of 10,998 vegetarians and non-vegetarians in the United Kingdom", *British Journal of Cancer*, 90 (2004): 118–121. https://www.nature.com/articles/6601441.

27 Ronald Schmid, *The Untold Story of Milk: Green Pastures, Contented Cows and Raw Dairy Foods* (Washington, DC: New Trends Publishing, 2003), 153.

28 "Arsenic in Your Food," *Consumer Reports Magazine*, November 2012, accessed March 8, 2015, http://www.consumerreports.org/cro /magazine/2012/11/arsenic-in-your-food/index.htm.

29 Daniel Auer, accessed 2013, http://www.doctorauer.com.

30 Allam AH, et al., "Atherosclerosis in Ancient Egyptian Mummies: the Horus Study," *JACC Cardiovascular Imaging*, 4, no. 4 (April 2011): 315–27, https://doi.org/10.1016/j.jcmg.2011.02.002.

31 Daniel Auer, accessed 2013, http://www.doctorauer.com.

32 Oak Creek Relief & Wellness Center, accessed May 2014, http://www.reliefandwellnesscenters.com.

33 Hadjivassiliou M, Sanders DS, Grunewald RA, Woodroofe N, Boscolo S, Aeschlimann D, "Gluten Sensitivity: From Gut to Brain," *Lancet Neurology*, 9, no. 3 (March 2010): 318–330.

34 Burk K, Bosch S, Muller CA, Melms A, Zuhlke C, Stern M, Besenthal I, Skalej M, Ruck P, Ferber S, Klockgether T, Dichgans J, "Sporadic Cerebellar Ataxia Associated with Gluten Sensitivity," *Brain*, 124, pt. 5 (May 2001): 1013–1019.

35 Hu WT, Murray JA, Greenaway MC, Parisi JE, Josephs KA, "Cognitive Impairment and Celiac Disease," *Archives of Neurology*, 63, no. 10 (October 2006): 1440–1446.

36 Borhani Haghighi A, Ansari N, Mokhtari M, Geramizadeh B, Lankarani KB, "Multiple Sclerosis and Gluten Sensitivity," *Clin Neurol Neurosurg*, 109, no. 8 (October 2007): 651–653.

37 Rashtak S, Rashtak S, Synder MR, Pittock SJ, Wu TT, Gandhi MJ, Murry JA, "Serology of Celiac Disease in Gluten-Sensitive Ataxia or Neuropathy: Role of Deamidated Gliadin Antibody," *J Neuroimmunol.*, 230, no. 1–2 (January 2011): 130–134. https://doi.org/10.1016/j.jneuroim.2010.09.024.

38 Volta U, De Giogio R, "Gluten Sensitivity: An Emerging Issue Behind Neurological Impairment?" *Lancet Neurol.* 9, no. 3 (March 2010): 233–235. https://doi.org/10.1016/S1474-4422(09)70357-6.

39 Savolainen H., "Sensory Ganglionopathy Due to Gluten Sensitivity," *Neurology* 77, no. 1 (July 2011): 87 [author reply]. http://doi.org/10.1212/WNL.0b013e318219a12d.

40 Ruuskanen A, Kaukinen K, Collin P, et al., "Gliadin Antibodies in Older Population and Neurological and Psychiatric Disorders," *Acta Neurol Scand.* 127, no. 1 (January 2013; epub April 12, 2012): 19–25. https://doi.org/10.1111/j.1600-0404.2012.01668.x.

41 Schlesinger I, Hering R, "Antigliadin Antibodies in Migraine Patients," *Cephalalgia*, 17, no. 6 (October 1997): 712.

42 Moccia M, Pellecchia MT, Erro R, et al., "Restless Legs Syndrome is a Common Feature of Adult Celiac Disease," *Mov Disord*, 25, no. 7, (May 2010): 877–881.

43 Datis Kharrazian, *Why Isn't My Brain Working?* (Carlsbad: Elephant Press, 2013), 134.

44 Fasano A, "CeliacD—How to Handle a Clinical Chameleon," *N Engl J Med.*, 348 (June 2003): 25. https://doi.org/10.1056/NEJMe030050.

45 Kamin DS, Furuta GT, "The Iceberg Cometh: Establishing the Prevalence of Celiac Disease in the United States and Finland," *Gastroenterology*, 126, no. 1 (January 2004): 359–361.

46 Corrao G, Corazza GR, Bagnardi V, et al., "Mortality in Patients with Coeliac Disease and Their Relatives: a Cohort Study," *Lancet,* 358, no. 9279 (August 2001): 356–361.

47 Green PHR, Alaedini A, Sander HW, Brannagan TH, Latovand N, Chin RL, "Mechanisms Underlying Celiac Disease and Its Neurologic Manifestations," *Cell Mol Life Sci.*, 62, no. 7–8 (April 2005): 791–799.

48 Ventura A, Magazzù G, Greco L, "Duration of Exposure to Gluten and Risk for Autoimmune Disorders in Patients with Celiac Disease," *Gastroenterology*, 117, no. 2 (August 1999): 297–303.

49 Corrao G, Corazza GR, Bagnardi V, et al., "Mortality in Patients with Coeliac Disease: a Cohort Study," *Lancet*, 358, no. 9279 (2001): 356–361.

50 Dairy Farming Today, accessed June 1, 2014, http://www.dairyfarmingtoday.org/Learn-More/FactsandFigures/Pages/FactsFigures.aspx.

51 Arola H, Tamm A, "Metabolism of Lactose in the Human Body," *Scandinavian Journal of Gastroenterology*, 202, suppl (1994): 21–25.

52 Share Care, accessed January 15, 2014, http://www.sharecare.com/health/lactose-intolerance/what-causes-lactose-intolerance.

53 Digestive Disease Center of the Hudson Valley, accessed February 13, 2014, http://www.digestivediseaseny.com/procedures/food-intolerances.

54 Vojdani A, Tarash, I. "Cross-Reaction Between Gliadin and Different Food and Tissue Antigens," *Food and Nutrition Sciences*, 4, no. 1 (January 2013): 20–32. doi:10.4236/fns.2013.41005. http://www.scirp.org/journal/fns.

55 Rebecca M. LaDronka, Samantha Ainsworth, Melinda J. Wilkins, Bo Norby, Todd M. Byrem, Paul C. Bartlett, "Prevalence of Bovine Leukemia Virus Antibodies in US Dairy Cattle," *Veterinary Medicine International*, 2018: article ID 5831278. Published online 2018 Nov 11. http://doi.org/10.1155/2018/5831278.

56 Feskanich D, Willett WC, Stampfer MJ, Colditz GA, "Milk, Dietary Calcium and Bone Fractures in Women: a 12-Year Prospective Study," *Am J Public Health*, 87, no. 6 (June 1997): 992–997. Accessed 2013, cited on everydayliving.com.

57 Virtanen SM, Räsänen L, Ylönen K, et al., "Early Introduction of Dairy Products Associated with Increased Risk of IDDM in Finnish Children.

The Childhood in Diabetes in Finland Study Group," *Diabetes*, 42, no. 12 (December 1993): 1786–1790.

58 Goldfarb MF, "Relation of Time of Introduction of Cow Milk Protein to an Infant and Risk of Type-1 Diabetes Mellitus," *J Proteome Res*, 7, no. 5 (May 2008): 2165–2167. http://doi.org/10.1021/pr800041d.

59 Berry CE, Hare JM, "Xanthine Oxidoreductase and Cardiovascular Disease: Molecular Mechanisms and Pathophysiological Implications," *J Physiol.*, 555, pt. 3 (2004): 589–606.

60 Malosse D, Perron H, Sasco A, Seigneurin JM, "Correlation Between Milk and Dairy Product Consumption and Multiple Sclerosis Prevalence: a Worldwide Study," *Neuroepidemiology*, 11, nos. 4–6 (1992): 304–312.

61 Jennifer Reid Holman, "Respiratory Symptoms Strongly Predict More Persistent Cow's Milk Allergy," *Medscape Medical News*, ACAAI 2006 Annual Meeting: Abstract 13 (November 2006).

62 Holman, "Respiratory Symptoms Predict Allergy."

63 William Sears, "Milk Allergies," askdrsears.com.

64 "Lactose Intolerance," website of the National Institute of Diabetes and Digestive and Kidney Diseases, http://digestive.niddk.nih.gov /ddiseases/pubs/lactoseintolerance/, http://www.niddk.nih.gov /health-information/digestive-diseases/lactose-intolerance.

65 Full petition: https://www.federalregister.gov/articles/2013/02/20/2013 -03835/flavored-milk-petition-to-amend-the-standard-of-identity-for -milk-and-17-additional-dairy-products.

66 Barrett JR, "The Science of Soy: What Do We Really Know?" *Environmental Health Perspectives*, 114, no. 6 (June 2006): A352–A358.

67 U.S. Food and Drug Administration, Code of Federal Regulations, Title 21, April 1, 2016. https://www.accessdata.fda.gov/scripts/cdrh/cfdocs /cfcfr/CFRSearch.cfm?fr=101.82.

68 US FDA CFR Title 21, April 1, 2016.

69 Kaayla Daniel, *The Whole Soy Story: The Dark Side of America's Favorite Health Food* (Washington, DC: New Trends Publishing, 2005), 266.

70 Daniel, *Whole Soy Story*, 147.

71 Konke L, "Could Eating Too Much Soy Be Bad for You?" accessed October 22, 2013, http://www.scientificamerican.com/article. cfm?id=soybean-fertility-hormone-isoflavones-genistein.

72 Fitzpatrick M, "Soy Formulas and the Effects of Isoflavones on the Thyroid," *New Zealand Med J*. 113, no. 1103 (2000): 24–26.

73 Daniel, *Whole Soy Story*.

74 Elliott SS, Keim NL, Stern JS, Teff K, Havel PJ, "Fructose, Weight Gain, and the Insulin Resistance Syndrome," *Am J Clin Nutr* 76, no. 5 (November 2002): 911–922. PMID 12399260.

75 Basciano H, Federico L, Adeli K, "Fructose, Insulin Resistance, and Metabolic Dyslipidemia," *Nutrition & Metabolism* 2, no. 5 (2005): 5. doi:10.1186/1743-7075-2-5. PMC 552336. PMID 15723702. http://doi.org/10.1093/ajcn/76.5.911.

76 Nancy Appleton. *Lick the Sugar Habit* (Santa Monica: Avery, 1996).

77 Johnson RJ, Segal MS, Sautin Y, et al., "Potential Role of Sugar (Fructose) in the Epidemic of Hypertension, Obesity and the Metabolic Syndrome, Diabetes, Kidney Disease, and Cardiovascular Disease," *Am J Clin Nutr*, 86, no. 4 (October 2007): 899–906.

78 Boyd DB, "Insulin and Cancer," *Integr Cancer Ther.*, 2, no. 4 (December 2003): 315–29.

79 Ludwig DS, Peterson KE, Gortmaker SL, "Relation Between Consumption of Sugar-Sweetened Drinks and Childhood Obesity: a Prospective, Observational Analysis," *Lancet*, 357, no. 9255 (February 2001): 505–8.

80 Stanhope KL, et al. "Consuming Fructose-Sweetened, Not Glucose-Sweetened, Beverages Increases Visceral Adiposity and Lipids and Decreases Insulin Sensitivity in Overweight/Obese Humans," *J Clin Invest.* 119, no. 5 (May 2009): 1322–34.

81 Page KA, et al. "Effects of Fructose vs Glucose on Regional Cerebral Blood Flow in Brain Regions Involved with Appetite and Reward Pathways," *JAMA*, 309, no. 1 (January 2013): 63–70. http://doi.org/10.1001/jama.2012.116975.

82 Skoog SM, Bharucha AE, "Dietary Fructose and Gastrointestinal Symptoms: a Review." *Am J Gastroenterol*, 99, no. 10 (2004): 2046–2050. http://doi.org/10.1111/j.1572-0241.2004.40266.x. PMID 15447771.

83 Beyer PL, Caviar EM, McCallum RW, "Fructose Intake at Current Levels in the United States May Cause Gastrointestinal Distress in Normal Adults," *J Am Diet Assoc* 105, no. 10 (2005): 1559–1566. doi:10.1016/j.jada.2005.07.002. PMID 16183355.

84 Lustig RB, "Fructose: Metabolic, Hedonic, and Societal Parallels with Ethanol," *J Am Diet Assoc.* 110, no. 9 (September 2010): 1307–1321.

85 Cheng CW, et al. "Prolonged Fasting Reduces IGF-1/PKA to Promote Hematopoietic-Stem-Cell-Based Regeneration and Reverse Immunosuppression," *Cell Stem Cell*, 14, no. 6 (June 2014): 810. http://doi.org/10.1016/j.stem.2014.04.014.

86 Reganold JP, Andrews PK, Reeve JR, et al., "Fruit and Soil Quality of Organic and Conventional Strawberry Agroecosystems." *PLOS One*, 5, no. 9 (September 2010) http://doi.org/10.1371/journal.pone.0012346.

87 Reaganold, "Fruit and Soil Quality," *PLOS One.*

88 International Scientific Association for Probiotics and Prebiotics, "Probiotics: A Consumer Guide for Making Smart Choices," PDF accessed from website of the ISAPPS, https://isappscience.org/clinicians/consumer-guidelines-probiotic/

89 Timothy Hand, Yasmine Belkaid, "Microbial Control of Regulatory and Effector T-Cell Responses in the Gut," *Curr Opin Immunol*, 22, no. 1 (February 2010): 63–72. http://doi.org/10.1016/j.coi.2010.01.008.

90 Wall R, Ross RP, Fitzgerald GF, Stanton C. "Fatty Acids from Fish: the Anti-Inflammatory Potential of Long-Chain Omega-3 Fatty Acids," *Nutr Rev*, 68, no. 5 (May 2010) 280–9. http://doi.org/10.1111/j.1753-4887.2010.00287.x.

91 Betiati Dda S, de Oliveira PF, Camargo Cde Q, Nunes EA, Trindade EB, "Effects of Omega-3 Fatty Acids on Regulatory T Cells in Hematologic Neoplasms," *Rev Bras Hematol Hemoter*, 35, no. 2 (2013): 119–125. http://doi.org/10.5581/1516-8484.20130033.

92 Cesarone MR, Belcaro G, Di Renzo A, et al., "Prevention of Influenza Episodes with Colostrum Compared with Vaccination in Healthy and High-Risk Cardiovascular Subjects: the Epidemiologic Study in San Valentino," *Clin Appl Thromb Hemost*, 13, no. 2 (April 2007): 130–136.

93 Hegde VL, Hegde S, Cravatt BF, Hofseth LF, Nagarkatti M, Nagarkatti PS. "Attenuation of Experimental Autoimmune Hepatitis by Exogenous and Endogenous Cannabinoids: Involvement of Regulatory T-Cells," *Mol Pharmacol*, 74, no. 1 (July 2008): 20–33. http://doi.org/10.1124/mol.108.047035.

94 Maresz K, Pryce G, Ponomarev ED, et al., "Direct Suppression of CNS Autoimmune Inflammation Via the Cannabinoid Receptor CB1 on Neurons and CB2 on Autoreactive T-cells," *Natural Med*, 13, no. 4 (April 2007): 492–497. http://doi.org/10.1038/nm1561.

95 Cianchi F, Papucci L, Schiavone N, et al., "Cannabinoid receptor activation induces apoptosis through tumor necrosis factor alpha-mediated ceramide de novo synthesis in colon cancer cells," *Clin Cancer Res*, 14, no.23 (December 2008): 7691–700, accessed 2013, http://clincancerres.aacrjournals.org/content/14/23/7691.long, http://doi.org/10.1158/1078-0432.CCR-08-0799.

96 Guy A. Cabral, Thomas J. Rogers, Aron H. Lichtman, "Turning Over a New Leaf: Cannabinoid and Endocannabinoid Modulation of Immune Function," *J Neuroimmune Pharmacol*, 10, no. 2 (June 2015); 193–203. http://doi.org10.1007/s11481-015-9615-z.

97 Fujita T, Sakurai K, "Efficacy of Glutamine-Enriched Enteral Nutrition in an Experimental Model of Mucosal Ulcerative Colitis," *Br J Surg*, 82, no. 6 (June 1995): 749–51.

98 Van der Hulst RRWJ, von Meyenfeldt MF, Deutz NEP, et al., "Glutamine and the Preservation of Gut Integrity," *Lancet*, 341, no. 8857 (May 1993): 1363–5.

99 Vogler BK, Ernst E. "Aloe Vera: a Systematic Review of Its Clinical Effectiveness," *Br J Gen Prac*, 49, no. 447 (October 1999): 823–828.

100 Boudreau MD, Beland FA, "An Evaluation of the Biological and Toxicological Properties of *Aloe barbadensis* (Miller), Aloe Vera," *J Environ Sci Health C Environ Carcinog Ecotoxicol Rev*, 24, no. 1 (Apr 2006); 103–54.

101 Gupta SK, Prakash J, Srivastava S, "Validation of Traditional Claim of Tulsi, *Ocimum sanctum Linn.* as a Medicinal Plant," *Indian J Exp Biol*, 40, no. 7 (July 2002): 765–73.

102 Uma Devi P, "Radioprotective, Anticarcinogenic and Antioxidant Properties of the Indian Holy Basil, *Ocimum sanctum* (Tulasi)," *Indian J Exp Biol*, 39, no. 3 (March 2001): 185–90.

103 Batmanghelidj F, *Your Body's Many Cries for Water; You're Not Sick; You're Thirsty: Don't Treat Thirst with Medications, 3rd ed.* (Global Health Solutions; 2008).

104 http://www.nhlbi.nih.gov/health/health-topics/topics/sdd/why.html. https://www.nhlbi.nih.gov/health-topics/sleep-deprivation-and -deficiency

105 Mandy Oaklander, "This Is Your Brain on 10 Years of Working the Night Shift," *Time Magazine* (November 4, 2014) http://time.com/3556130 /night-shift-brain-work-health.

Bibliography

Appleton, Nancy. *Lick the Sugar Habit: Sugar Addiction Upsets Your Whole Body Chemistry.* Santa Monica, CA: Avery, 1996.

Batmanghelidj, Fereydoon. *Your Body's Many Cries for Water: You're Not Sick; You're Thirsty: Don't Treat Thirst with Medications*, 3rd ed. San Francisco, CA: Global Health Solutions, 2008.

Campbell, T. Colin. *The China Study: Startling Implications for Diet, Weight Loss, and Long-Term Health.* Dallas, TX: BenBella Books, 2005.

Clark, Daniel, and Kaye Wyatt. *Colostrum: Life's First Food.* Salt Lake City, UT: Center Nutritional Research House Publications, 1996.

Cordain, Loren. *The Paleo Diet: Lose Weight and Get Healthy by Eating the Foods You Were Designed to Eat.* Boston, MA: Houghton Mifflin Harcourt, 2002.

Daniel, Kaayla T. *The Whole Soy Story: The Dark Side of America's Favorite Health Food.* Washington, DC: New Trends Publishing, 2005.

Dispenza, Joe. *Breaking the Habit of Being Yourself: How to Lose Your Mind and Create a New One.* Carlsbad, CA: Hay House, 2012.

Dufty, William. *Sugar Blues.* New York: Warner Books, 1976.

Erasmus, Udo. *Fats that Heal, Fats that Kill: the Complete Guide to Fats, Oils, Cholesterol and Human Health.* Alamo, CA: Alive Book Publishing, 2010.

Gedgaudas, Nora T. *Primal Body, Primal Mind: Beyond the Paleo Diet for Total Health and a Longer Life.* Rochester, VT: Healing Arts Press, 2011.

Gershon, Michael D. *The Second Brain: The Scientific Basis of Gut Instinct and a Groundbreaking New Understanding of Nervous Disorders of the Stomach and Intestines.* New York: HarperCollins, 1999.

Graham, Gray, Deborah Kesten, Larry Scherwitz. *Pottenger's Prophecy: How Food Resets Genes for Wellness or Illness.* Tumwater, WA: Destiny Health Publishing, 2011.

Keith, Lierre. *The Vegetarian Myth: Food, Justice, and Sustainability.* Oakland, CA: PM Press, 2009.

Kharrazian, Datis. *Why Isn't My Brain Working?: A Revolutionary Understanding of Brain Decline and Effective Strategies to Recover Your Brain's Health.* Carlsbad, CA: Elephant Press, 2013.

Lipton, Bruce. *The Biology of Belief: Unleashing the Power of Consciousness, Matter & Miracles.* Carlsbad, CA: Hay House, 2015.

Ottolenghi, Yotam, and Sami Tamimi. *Jerusalem: A Cookbook.* Berkeley, CA: Ten Speed Press, 2012.

Phinney, Stephen D., and Jeff S. Volek. *The Art and Science of Low Carbohydrate Living.* Miami, FL: Beyond Obesity, 2011.

———. *The Art and Science of Low Carbohydrate Performance.* Miami, FL: Beyond Obesity, 2012.

Price, Weston. *Nutrition and Physical Degeneration.* Lemon Grove, CA: Price-Pottenger Nutrition Foundation, 2009.

Rogers, Matthew, and Tiziana Alipo Tamborra. *Sweet Gratitude: A New World of Raw Desserts.* Berkeley, CA: North Atlantic Books, 2012.

Schmid, Ronald. *The Untold Story of Milk: Green Pastures, Contented Cows and Raw Dairy Foods.* Washington, DC: New Trends Publishing, 2003.

Sisson, Mark, and Jennifer Meier. *The Primal Blueprint Cookbook: Primal, Low Carb, Paleo, Grain-Free, Dairy-Free and Gluten-Free.* Malibu, CA: Primal Nutrition, 2010.

Smith, Jeffrey. *Genetic Roulette: The Gamble of Our Lives.* DVD. Directed by Jeffrey Smith. Fairfield, CA: Institute for Responsible Technology, 2012.

Upledger, John. *Your Inner Physician and You: CranioSacral Therapy and Somatoemotional Release.* Berkeley, CA: North Atlantic Books, 1997.

Weissman, Darren. *Awakening to the Secret Code of Your Mind: Your Mind's Journey to Inner Peace.* Carlsbad, CA: Hay House, 2010.

Acknowledgments

I want to thank the many pioneers in the field of health and wellness who have shared their gifts with the world and allowed me to use their wisdom and science to alleviate suffering in some way. I offer thanks to some of the most knowledgeable healthcare providers and spiritual teachers in the world for the high honor it has been to meet many of you and learn from you all: Dr. Dietrich Klinghardt, Dr. Datis Kharrazian, Dr. Aristo Vojdani, Dr. Thomas O'Bryan, Dr. Nazanin Kimiai, Dr. Darren Weissman, Dr. Thomas Rau, Dr. Konrad Wertmann, Dr. Joseph Mercola, Dr. Bruce Lipton, Gregg Braden, Dr. Kari Vernon, Dr. Thomas Culleton, Vanessa Morgan, Dr. Christopher Hansard, Dr. John Upledger, Karma Sungrap Ngedon Tenpa Gyaltsen, the 7th Dzogchen Ponlop Rinpoche, Khenchen Tsültrim Gyamtso Rinpoche, Pema Chodron, and Tenzin Gyatso, the 14th Dalai Lama.

Thanks to Shane McDermott, my dear Integrally-informed friend, for all your time and heart-to-heart talks, leaving me in deep contemplation, tears, and laughter. Thanks to my Thrive family, especially Jesse Koren and Sharla Jacobs, for the endless encouragement, practical business support, and frequent reminders that mistakes are sexy. Thanks to my Sedona family— Charly Wells, KrissKringle Sprinkle, and Mary Mulcahy—for broadening my awareness.

I want to thank the thousands of patients I have worked with throughout the years and dozens of friends and family members who have taught me more than words can express.

Thanks to my beloved husband and wordsmith genius for his editing skill and to my editing team, Cate Montana, and publicist Gail Torr.

Thanks to Cyrex Labs and Principal Labs for making tests available that are changing the world . . . and how we live in it.

Index

Page numbers in **boldface** indicate the location of the primary discussion of the term.

FOOD LIST

RECIPES

About the Author

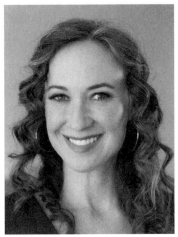

Photo by Ben Hoffman

Kristin Grayce McGary LAc., MAc., CFMP®, CST-T, CLP is an internationally recognized authority on autoimmunity, functional blood chemistry analysis, thyroid and gut health, food as medicine, and integrating mind, body, and spirit in healthcare. A health and lifestyle alchemist, author, and speaker, she weaves more than 22 years of experience, education, and wisdom into compassion to empower you to heal on all levels. Kristin Grayce lives in Boulder, Colorado.

For more information see: *www.kristingraycemcgary.com*